PATHWAYS TO A CENTERED BODY

ALSO BY DONNA FARHI

The Breathing Book

Yoga, Mind, Body & Spirit: A Return to Wholeness

Bringing Yoga to Life: The Everyday Practice of Enlightened Living

Teaching Yoga: Exploring the Teacher-Student Relationship

Pathways to a Centered Body

GENTLE YOGA THERAPY FOR CORE STABILITY,
HEALING BACK PAIN, AND MOVING WITH EASE

Donna Farhi and Leila Stuart

Illustrations by Sonya Rooney

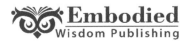
Embodied
Wisdom Publishing

Illustrations by Sonya Rooney, Christchurch, New Zealand.
Photographs by Murray Irwin, Mannering & Associates Ltd, Christchurch, New Zealand
Cover and Text Design by Gopa & Ted2, Inc.
www.gopated2inc.com
Printed in China.

26 25 24 23 22   10 9 8 7 6 5 4 3 2

ISBN	978-0-473-58600-3
Title	Pathways to a Centered Body: Gentle Yoga Therapy for Core Stability, Healing Back Pain, and Moving with Ease.
Authors	Donna Farhi and Leila Stuart
Format	Softcover
Publication Date	01/2022 | Second edition

Disclaimer

The information provided in this book is not intended as a substitute for the medical advice of physicians or other qualified health professionals. This book is not intended to diagnose or treat any medical condition, but rather to describe one approach to healthy movement function. The reader is advised to regularly consult a physician in health matters, particularly for diagnosis or treatment of any medical condition and before undertaking the practices in this book. The publisher and authors are not liable for any injuries, damages, or negative consequences allegedly arising from reading or using information in this book.

Table of Contents

Introduction

I N RECENT TIMES, core fitness has become a catch phrase for a multitude of physical fitness regimens geared toward firming and strengthening the core muscles of the body. With increasingly sedentary lifestyles and the accompanying epidemic of obesity that has followed, core fitness has become almost synonymous with losing weight and regaining a trim, flat, and defined waistline. For some of us, improving core strength and stability offers the promise of alleviation of back pain, allowing us to move through the day with less discomfort or to resume activities, such as running or playing golf. For athletes, dancers, and practitioners of Yoga, having a strong core may translate into having more refined control of the body and the ability to do breathtakingly virtuosic movements. But what do we really mean when we talk about having a strong core? Why is it important to center the pelvis and to have stability in the core muscles of the body? And what muscles are we actually referring to when we speak of the core?

As practitioners and teachers of Yoga with more than five decades of combined experience, we have observed this trend and believe many of the approaches to core fitness, and the movement disciplines catering to its pursuit, often have limited efficacy because they neglect to address the deeper foundation muscles that form the scaffolding for a truly centered pelvis and upright spine. Furthermore, when these deeper core muscles are weak, tight, or unbalanced, strengthening the more superficial muscles of the body may serve only to mask and even accentuate the preexisting body imbalance. The "abs of steel" that have become so much a part of our cultural obsession with the body beautiful actually can *contribute to* ongoing back pain, shallow breathing, and movement dysfunction. On the other end of the spectrum, we also have seen a worldwide epidemic of hypermobile Yoga practitioners who complain of chronic discomfort and reoccurring injuries. Most of these injuries are the result of the pursuit of extreme flexibility without building a foundation of strong and stable musculature.

THE CORE AND THE PSOAS

This book distinguishes between primary core muscles and secondary core muscles (more about these later). The primary core muscle we'll be exploring is the psoas muscle (pronounced *so-az* with a silent p), or more correctly, the iliopsoas muscle complex (Illustration 1, page 8). Defined as a "deep" abdominal muscle, the psoas lies in the back or posterior of the abdominal wall and cannot be readily palpated.[1] The structure of the psoas is exceedingly complex, and some of the finest anatomists, clinicians, and somatic practitioners have differing views about the movement function of the psoas. These three factors—that is, its deeply buried position, difficulty in palpation, and controversy over its function—go a long way toward explaining why the psoas often is omitted from discussions about core stability and why it has been given so little mention in movement practices and, indeed, in many clinical and therapeutic modalities.

Because of its unique central position and function, the psoas has a multidimensional influence on our experience of stability, strength, ease, and coordination. From their origin in the back of the body, the left and right psoas muscles are anchored to the lumbar spine. The muscles swoop diagonally forward to the front of the pelvis and then make a backward detour to attach to the inside of the thigh bones. Given their distinct angles of pull on the spinal column, pelvis, and hip bones, the psoas are a key determinant of the position of the pelvis and have a profound effect on the functional stability of the body. For this reason, we believe balancing this muscle should *precede* strengthening of the secondary core muscles. Once the psoas is acting as the primary initiator of core movement, the other secondary core muscles contract in concert to achieve optimal strength and function.

Dr. Janet Travell, coauthor of the classic trigger point manual *Myofascial Pain and Dysfunction*

calls the psoas "the hidden prankster" because of its deeply concealed and difficult-to-access location, and its ability to cause pain that is commonly attributed to other dysfunctions.[2] A more apt term might be "hidden treasure" because when patiently released and balanced through awareness and gentle exercises, the psoas can facilitate profound healing and relief from a multitude of discomforts and conditions.

As teachers who have worked with hundreds of Yoga students from all walks of life, it has been our experience that when the psoas does its job in centering the pelvis and stabilizing the lumbar spine, it minimizes the effort of more external muscles. When the psoas is functioning optimally, the pelvis and lumbar spine will be in a neutral position and stabilized from deep within, creating an experience of effortless verticality that is expressed in graceful integrated posture and movement. This physical centeredness can liberate energetic resources and promote a harmonious flow of energy and breath in the body (known as *prana* within the Yoga tradition or *qi* or *chi* in martial arts traditions). Creating core balance also may help you to feel more emotionally secure and able to meet previously overwhelming situations with robustness and resilience. Knowing how to hold your ground may correlate to a powerful psychodynamic stability and imperturbability that gives skillfulness to your speech and action. However we quantify the meaning of core, being centered in the present moment can help us to live from our deepest values and to focus on what ultimately matters.

As Yoga teachers, we are well aware that functionally integrated movement can never be reduced to one muscle. Rather, full movement capacity is the net result of the individual parts of the body working together in a synergistic relationship. So let us be clear at the beginning: we don't see a competent psoas muscle as a somatic panacea for all that ails you. That would be too simplistic. But we do believe its role in providing an easeful experience in the body has been little understood, and when the psoas is given even a modicum of attention, the results are often quite remarkable. We also believe that many of the methods for releasing the psoas are unnecessarily painful and can contribute to this deep muscle becoming even more contracted. We have seen students with conditions such as chronic lower back pain and unrelenting sciatica, as well as those with long-standing sacroiliac discomfort, feel immediate relief from simple exercises that can be practiced in as few as 5–10 minutes. When you consider that most of the exercises in this book require little more than an inexpensive Muscle Release Ball and a few blankets, that's a small investment for a big result.[3] The accessibility of these techniques can be especially significant for dancers, Yoga practitioners, athletes, and others who may not be able to afford regular bodywork and therefore are highly motivated to manage their own self-care. Many of our students have been surprised to discover that it is possible to correct longstanding conditions, such as hyperlordosis (an accentuation of the lumbar curve), with exercises and supported releases that, when practiced correctly, are without exception *pain free*.

Six-Step Protocol

To fully benefit from this work, we have developed a step-by-step protocol that will build both your cognitive and experiential understanding of the psoas as well as how to access its support. The six steps in this journey are as follows:

1. Find It: It's difficult to change any part of the body if you don't know where it is, what it looks like, and how it functions. The field of experiential anatomy (as opposed to purely theoretical study) uses visual imagery of anatomical structure combined with awareness through movement to give

a *felt* experience of body structure. We'll begin this process by learning about the anatomy of the iliopsoas complex followed by some simple techniques for tracing and locating the muscle. This information is in Chapters Two and Three.

2. Soften and Hydrate It: We believe that stretching any muscle before it has been warmed, softened, and hydrated can contribute to further defensive binding and potential injury of muscle tissue. Unfortunately, many Yoga methodologies do not include sufficient conditioning movements and proceed immediately to static postures that pull on the muscles. Consider how moistened pastry dough can be rolled paper thin, whereas dry crumbly dough cracks and crumbles even with the slightest pressure, and you get the idea. We'll introduce you to some effective techniques that use pulsing and oscillatory movement to generate circulation of fluid through muscle, fascia, and organ tissue. This information is in Chapter Four.

3. Release and Lengthen It: Incorporating the support of full diaphragmatic breathing, we learn to release and lengthen muscles as a dynamic process of uncoiling followed by slight retraction. Gentle stretching and releasing can further hydrate muscle and fascial tissue. In this section, you'll learn a veritable treasure trove of both active and passive release positions and techniques for gently and painlessly releasing the psoas muscles. This information is in Chapter Five.

4. Balance It: When significant asymmetries exist between the right and left sides of the body, it makes sense to address these imbalances *before* strengthening work, otherwise you risk the possibility of simply reinforcing your existing imbalance. Many of the techniques shown in this section can be helpful for those with spinal scoliosis (lateral curvature of the spine) and for one-sided spinal discomfort. This information is in Chapter Six.

5. Strengthen It: This section will teach you to consciously activate the psoas. We will introduce

you to the secondary core muscles and explain why coactivation of these muscles is such an important component of spinal health and optimal movement function. Then, the secondary core muscles can work synergistically with the psoas to support dynamic movement. This information is in Chapter Seven.

6. Move from It: This section offers you some suggestions for how to heighten awareness of psoas integration while practicing Yoga postures. Although our emphasis is on Yoga, many of these postures are practiced by athletes, dancers, and somatic practitioners in modified forms. We have also included a special section on how to safely mobilize your hip joints without compromising sacroiliac stability. You'll find this information in Chapter Eight. Sustaining good posture and movement alignment in all everyday activities reduces the allostatic loading (otherwise known as "wear and tear") on other body structures, such as knees, hips, and spine, promoting lifelong healthy joints, ligaments, and tendons. This information is in Chapter Nine.

A BROADER DEFINITION OF CORE STABILITY: A KOSHIC PERSPECTIVE

Before we begin learning about the anatomy of the psoas, this introduction would be sorely lacking without at least some mention of the broader definition of core stability. While the subject of this book is primarily the physical dimension of core stability, we recognize the core *as a multifaceted experience of self that is centered in the present.* From a Yogic viewpoint, the visible physical body is only one dimension of our total embodiment. When we watch an airplane take off, we see the obvious external structure of the plane that is essentially an aluminum cylinder. Yet we're equally aware that what we can see (the visible plane) is not what gets the plane off the ground. The complex hidden wiring of electrical and com-

puter systems, the engine and jet fuel, and the decisions of the pilot make the plane airborne yet are largely invisible to us. Similarly, our physical structure contains muscles, bones, connective tissue, internal organs, and body fluids, but a larger intelligence orchestrates these raw elements. In the Yogic tradition, we recognize that these invisible elements that operate on the level of the energetic, emotional, mental, and spiritual planes are all interwoven. What Yogis have known for centuries is now being scientifically backed by the discovery that our mind and emotions have a profound effect on our physical body. Conversely, the state of our physical body and health can have both positive and negative consequences on our mental and emotional state, as well as our ability to function in the world.

Although a thorough discussion is outside the scope of this book, we have outlined the geographic mapping of the body from a Yogic perspective and how core stability may be interpreted through this lens. In the Yogic paradigm, the body consists of different sheaths or *koshas*, which range from the gross experience of our physical structure, such as our muscles and bones, to subtler dimensions of embodiment, such as the flow of breath or a persistent pattern of thought or negative self-belief. Although you can't measure your thoughts and emotions with calipers, you know how deeply unsettling it can be to move through the day literally "off-balance" because your clear thinking has been eclipsed by a strong emotion such as anger or fear. Similarly, having a mental habit of always "being ahead of yourself" can have you sitting on the edge of your seat, pelvis tipped forward in anticipation of the next moment. The following *koshas* listed below may give you a broader perspective of what it means to find and sustain a sense of your true center.

1. Physical Body (*Annamaya Kosha*)
Structural Core Stability is defined as the ability to center your body in a clear relationship to ground,

gravity, and space. Bringing awareness to the core structures of the body can assist in the synergistic activation of both primary and secondary core muscles. Your body is then able to organize itself around a *fluidly stable* and responsive core. This supports you in your ability to transfer and direct force from the feet and legs up into the pelvis and through the spine into space and to mediate the force of gravity coming down through your body with minimal stress through your structure. The practices and inquiries in this book can help you to build structural core stability. Working with your physical body can become a doorway to deeper aspects of your self.

2. Energetic Body (*Pranamaya Kosha*)

Energetic Core Stability is defined as having a steady, reliable supply of energy to support daily activity. This is not the agitated energy that arises from stimulants such as sugar, caffeine, or alcohol, but a calm vibrant energy that is the result of a well-nourished body and the ability to settle into your center. Eastern traditions call this energetic center the *hara* or *tan dien* and both finding and learning to move from this potent center is a lifelong process.[4] In Western science, we refer to this center of intelligence as the "abdominal brain" or enteric nervous system, known colloquially as our "gut instinct."[5,6,7] The enteric nervous system of the gut constitutes an independent brain that is in an ongoing communication with the rest of the body.

In the Yogic tradition, the energetic body is understood as *prana* or life force, the mysterious animating force that orchestrates all the self-regulatory functions of the body, such as the movement of the blood, digestion of food, and elimination of waste. Prana underlies the support for the microcirculation of oxygen and nutrients at a cellular level and is expressed in full-body breathing through the movements of external respiration. These different roads all lead to the same destination: a deep navel center acting as a "Grand Central Station," coordinating impulses as they move in to and out of a firm center to each of the six limbs (the head, tail, two arms, and two legs). When energetic centeredness is mastered, even the smallest gesture appears to be orchestrated from the vital center, as can be witnessed in the movement of any great athlete, dancer, or martial artist. Although not all of us can become masters, anyone willing to invest a little time and energy can attain better posture and more grace in their movement.

The psoas muscles are the primary physical scaffolding supporting the energetic center. When you establish a stable structure with the help of the psoas, prana can circulate freely throughout your body. Movement that is initiated from your core is more efficient and requires less energy, which leaves more energy for you to enjoy your life.

3. Body of Feeling and Emotion (*Manamaya Kosha*)

Emotional Core Stability is defined as acquiring the ability to feel a broad range of emotions without losing a sense of a stable unchanging center. Cultivating emotional stability involves learning to welcome, meet, and greet your feelings and emotions through a neutral witnessing process that neither suppresses emotions nor inappropriately vents or expresses these emotions in a way that causes harm to others. Through this process, you learn to view your feelings and emotions as messengers offering valuable information about your experience, without eclipsing an awareness of the unchanging Self. Far from creating a cold-hearted detachment, being able to disidentify with emotions allows you to register your experience in high resolution without shutting down or becoming overwhelmed. This can increase your ability to remain centered and present for others who may be in the throes of their own strong emotional experience.

The psoas can be viewed as a repository of the instinctual emotions of the abdominal brain. Working tenderly with the psoas can sometimes unleash these emotions, but at the same time, it can provide access to the strength and innate wisdom necessary for the healing journey toward emotional wholeness.

4. Body of Thought (*Vijyanamaya Kosha*)

Mental Core Stability is the ability to establish and sustain the practice of *pratyahara*. Pratyahara is a Sanskrit term that refers to the restoration of the senses to their fullest function, whereby you begin to notice the unchanging ground from which experience arises. To be truly centered is to have a simultaneous awareness of both the changing patterns of your mind and the unchanging ground of consciousness. Balancing your mental process includes identifying and compassionately looking at the tendencies, habits, and programming that consistently draw you out of your core and prevent the emergence of your deep inner wisdom. Such presence of mind allows you to respond to each situation perfectly and appropriately.

The psoas can register the mental programming and metaphors with which we live, often resulting in excessive muscular tension. For example, if you live with a belief system that no one can be trusted, your vigilance will be embodied as tension in the psoas and other muscles of your body. When the psoas is hydrated and balanced, it can be used as a reliable physical tool to tap into the stillness that underlies and contains all thoughts, feelings, and emotions. It may help to establish a sense of being seated in your Self, accessing and relying on your authentic power and wisdom.

5. Body of Liberation (*Anandamaya Kosha*)

Spiritual Core Stability is about having a connection to your core purpose or *dharma* and truthfully maintaining a faithful allegiance to your unique life path. When you live with a sense of connectedness and intimacy with the world and others, ultimately there is no center and no periphery, no you or me, only an indivisible oneness. Working with the psoas can help you to have a felt sense of connectedness within yourself that can overflow into your relationships in the outer world. The physical stability that results from balancing the psoas can even result in feelings of greater connectedness.

One of the most tangible and immediate ways to begin the process of centering yourself is through and in the body. Because each kosha is inextricably linked to all the others, centering the physical body is one of the simplest and most immediate ways of balancing the other koshas. The psoas can function as a "touchstone" for accessing and balancing all the koshas.

Ultimately, it does not matter which door you choose to walk through while in the process of developing a better sense of center, but we encourage you to return again and again to your body as a reference point. Then, as you explore the many experiential inquiries and exercises in this book, take a little time to notice whether the structural work you have done has evoked any change in how you feel energetically, emotionally, mentally, and even spiritually. We call this observational process "body weather reading," and we encourage you to use this practice not only during and after you complete an exercise in this book, but also frequently throughout your busy day. Learning to recognize when you've moved away from center is the first step in finding your way back.

BODY WEATHER READING: THE IMPORTANCE OF BASELINE PERCEPTION

If you've ever gone for a walk in a large botanical park, you will be familiar with the maps posted at the entranceways with red arrows declaring "you are here." Because unless you know the point from which you are starting, it's impossible to navigate to where you want to go. Similarly, by doing a little body weather reading at the beginning of each practice session and noting how you are feeling, you then will be able to appreciate any changes that occur as a result of your practice. This process can be especially important when you are trying to ascertain which practices are most helpful in ameliorating discomfort and healing injuries.

Before you begin a practice session, take a little time (walking, standing, sitting, or lying down) to check in with your self. Using the koshas can be a handy framework for structuring your observations:

- How do you feel in your physical structure? Note any areas of tension or discomfort.

- What kind of energy level do you have today? Is your breath rhythmic?

- Are you aware of any particular feelings or emotions that are visiting today? If so, can you identify the nature of these visitors?

- Were your spirits high or low this morning? Reflect back to when you woke up.

After you practice an inquiry or exercise, take a few minutes to reflect again: has there been any physical change? If so, can you define it? If you began your session feeling depleted and fatigued, have your energy levels improved? If you began the session feeling anxious and unsettled, do you now feel more grounded? When you come up to standing at the end of each session and begin to move about your day, has your practice made a qualitative difference to the way you are operating in the world? It is through this careful observation and inquiry that you can come to know how to center yourself and to sustain that centeredness even as you step out into the world.

❖ How to Use This Book

To understand the rationale of many of the exercises and inquiries in this book it will be helpful to read the next chapter on the anatomy of the psoas. If, however, you feel intimidated by the subject of anatomy, there's no harm in skipping this chapter and moving directly to the practices in the chapters that follow. Or, if you want to glean the most important anatomical points, you can read the *Key Concepts* summarized at the end of each section. Just looking at the pictures or reading the key concepts can offer valuable insights. Once you've experienced some of the benefits of the practices, you may become curious about why the exercises are so effective and feel encouraged to take a peek at the anatomy.

If you have an existing Yoga practice, Pilates routine, or other fitness regimen, consider adding one or two exercises to your routine. Take some time to trial those exercises, which will make it easier to discern whether a specific exercise is of benefit to you. Once you become familiar with those practices, explore a new one. Feel free to pick and choose those practices that feel relevant to your goals, but note that our protocol has a logical progression and the exercises have been sequenced accordingly. Eventually, you will develop a repertoire of practices that you can use to meet your personal needs—whether to release a tight back, open your body after sitting at your desk, or strengthen your core to prepare for a challenging athletic event. ❖

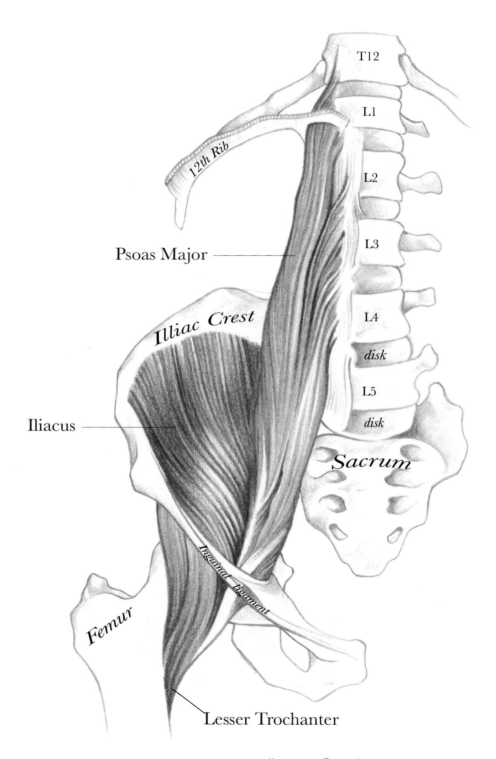

T12

L1

L2

L3

L4

disk

L5

disk

Sacrum

12th Rib

Psoas Major

Illiac Crest

Iliacus

Inguinal Ligament

Femur

Lesser Trochanter

ILLUSTRATION 1: Iliopsoas Complex

CHAPTER 2

The Anatomy of the Psoas

W E WANT TO tempt you to dive wholeheartedly into this chapter on the anatomy of the psoas by first revealing some of the amazing functions of this muscle. The effort that you put into studying the anatomy (or structure) and the kinesiology (the movement function) of this phenomenal muscle will give you a strong foundation to fully appreciate the broad-ranging capacities of the psoas. Understanding this anatomy also will give you crucial insights into the way the exercises offered in this book will work to release, balance, or strengthen the core body.

MULTIPLE FUNCTIONS OF THE PSOAS

The psoas carries out myriad functions and is truly a Yogic muscle as it serves to unify the body into a cohesive whole (Illustration 1).

The psoas creates a bridge by linking the following (Illustration 2):
- The upper body to the lower body
- The core to the periphery
- The back body to the front body
- The axial skeleton (spine and pelvis) to the appendicular skeleton (legs and arms)[1]

The psoas also has multiple functions:
- Central body support
- Lumbar stabilizer
- Regional muscular support for stabilizing the sacroiliac joint[2]
- Core initiator of movement
- Medium for effortless hip flexion and walking

The psoas can have a profound influence on the following:
- Full diaphragmatic breathing
- Healthy organ function
- Balancing the nervous system
- Psychological stability and resiliency

9

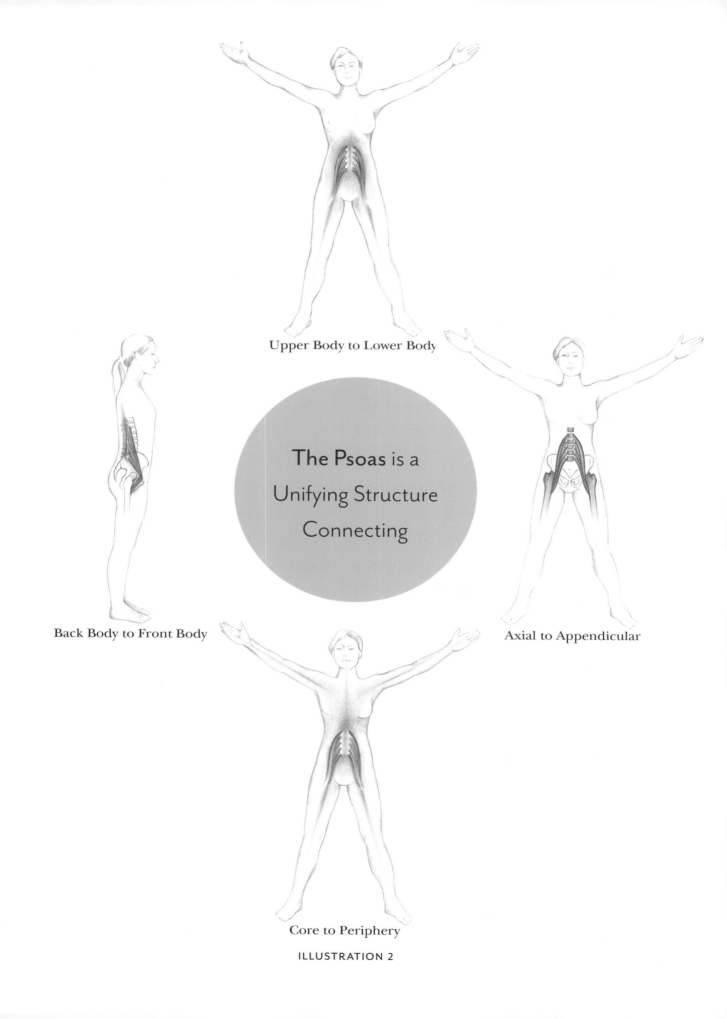

Upper Body to Lower Body

Back Body to Front Body

The Psoas is a
Unifying Structure
Connecting

Axial to Appendicular

Core to Periphery

ILLUSTRATION 2

❖ Helpful Anatomical Terms

Anterior refers to a structure in front of another structure in the body.

Posterior refers to a structure in back of another structure in the body.

Superior refers to a structure closer to the head than another structure in the body.

Inferior refers to a structure closer to the feet than another structure in the body.

Medial refers to a structure closer to the midline than another structure in the body.

Lateral refers to a structure farther away from the midline than another structure in the body.

Unilateral refers to a structure, action, or aspect that occurs on one side of the body only.

Bilateral refers to a structure, action, or aspect that occurs on both sides of the body simultaneously.

Flexion in the spine refers to bending forward. In other joints or body parts, it refers to two body parts moving closer together and decreasing the angle between them (e.g., in elbow flexion the forearm and upper arm come closer together).

Extension in the spine refers to bending backward and in other joints or body parts refers to two body parts moving away from each other and increasing the angle between them (e.g., in elbow extension the forearm and upper arm move further apart).

Lateral Flexion refers to bending a body part to the side.

Rotation refers to twisting or pivoting a part of the body.

Neutral Spinal Curves occur when the cervical, thoracic, and lumbar curves are balanced over a stable pelvis so that the spinal vertebrae have maximum space between them. A neutral lumbar curve is optimal in both standing alignment and functional movement to efficiently transfer force from the spine to the pelvis and legs.

Fascia traditionally is defined as the connective tissue primarily composed of collagen that forms sheaths or bands beneath the skin to attach, stabilize, enclose, and separate muscles and other internal organs. This definition currently is being broadened by findings in scientific and research circles to suggest that "all the collagenous-based soft tissues in the body, including the cells that create and maintain that network of extracellular matrix" come under the designation of fascia.[3] It may be helpful to imagine the fascia as a three-dimensional web connecting the entire body. A snag or thickening of fibers in one area of the web can have far-reaching consequences throughout the whole fabric of the body.

Ideokinesis is a form of somatic education that first came to prominence in the 1930s, using anatomically based, creative visual imagery to evoke conscious and refined neuromuscular coordination. "Ideo" means idea and "kinesis" refers to movement.

Intervertebral Disks are positioned between the vertebrae of the spine and consist of a tough outer layer called the annulus fibrosus and a soft jelly-like center called the nucleus pulposus. The intervertebral disks act as spacers and shock absorbers: loading weight compresses the disks, and when released, they regain their original shape. Chronic stress caused by overloading the spine, poor posture, or dysfunctional movement patterns (especially repetitive forward, backward, and twisting motions) can weaken the annulus and compromise the central position of the nucleus. In extreme cases, this can lead to disk herniation, whereby the annulus is completely ruptured and the gel of the nucleus leaks out. This can put pressure on the surrounding nerves and can cause severe pain. The malleable disks also contribute to spinal movement and maintenance of the spinal curves. Imagine how little our spine would move without the ability of the disks to stretch and compress.

Somatic refers to practices and approaches to embodiment that invite sensing, feeling, and acting from one's own sensory awareness. Thomas Hanna, Ph.D. (1928–1990) coined the word "somatics" in 1976 to name the approaches to mind–body integration where the body is experienced from within. "Soma" is a Greek word for the living body. ❖

❖ Psoas as Filet Mignon

To get a fuller appreciation of the sheer heft of the psoas muscles, the next time you are at the supermarket, pick up an entire filet mignon. Although humans certainly are not as large as cattle, seeing the size and feeling the weight of this muscle may give you a better sense of the substantial bulk of your own psoas muscles. Cut in cross-section, the many muscle bundles of the psoas are clearly delineated by the white envelopes of fascia. ❖

THE ILIOPSOAS COMPLEX

Although the three muscles in what is commonly referred to as the iliopsoas complex (psoas major, psoas minor, and iliacus) often are grouped together, each muscle has an individual identity and function. The Latin word *psoa* means "muscle of the loins" and in cattle is the tender filet mignon cut. In the upright human, the psoas muscle functions as a support structure, and as we'll soon see, it probably is not very tender in most people.

The largest muscle of the iliopsoas complex, the psoas major is approximately 41 centimeters long (16 inches) and is a thick triangular-shaped muscle that connects the spine to the legs. The psoas major is divided into two parts. The superficial portion arises from the sides of the 12th thoracic and the 1st–5th lumbar vertebrae, as well as the 1st–4th intervertebral disks. The deep portion arises from the transverse processes of the 1st–5th lumbar vertebrae (Illustration 3).

The psoas major journeys from its origin on the

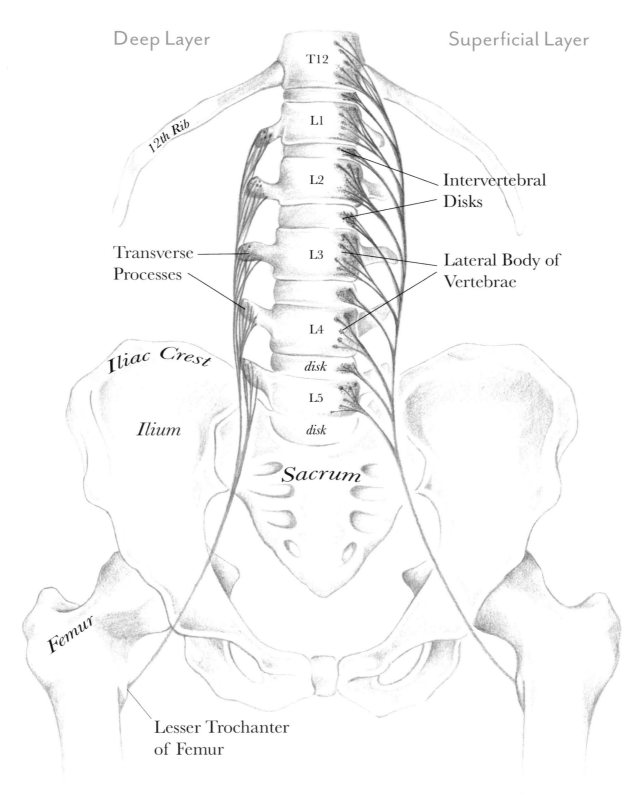

Deep Layer

Superficial Layer

T12

L1

L2

12th Rib

Intervertebral
Disks

Transverse
Processes

L3

Lateral Body of
Vertebrae

L4

disk

Iliac Crest

L5

disk

Ilium

Sacrum

Femur

Lesser Trochanter
of Femur

ILLUSTRATION 3:
Psoas Major Origins to Insertion

spine diagonally forward and laterally over the pubic bone and then dives backward to attach to the inside of the femur by a shared tendinous insertion with the iliacus (Illustration 1). Mechanically, this spatial arrangement allows the psoas to function as a pulley system that significantly increases the strength of the psoas.

The psoas minor is present in less than 50 percent of individuals. It connects the spine to the pelvis and may have been more relevant to four-legged creatures, which may explain the gradual evolutionary disappearance of this muscle in two-legged humans (Illustration 4).[4]

When present, it arises from the 12th thoracic and 1st lumbar vertebrae and attaches to the rim of the pubic bone via a long, thin tendon. The psoas minor helps to maintain the horizontal alignment of the pelvis. Contraction of the psoas minor can contribute to posterior rotation of the pelvis (as when you tuck the tailbone under) and lumbar flexion (a flattening of the lumbar curve).

In most quadrupeds, the psoas major does not touch the pelvis but instead connects directly from the spine to the femur (Illustration 5A). Evolution to upright standing has put a different stress on the psoas, requiring it to bend around the pelvis before detouring to the femur (Illustration 5B). The psoas is under considerable tension just in the simple act of standing or lying down with the legs straight. Thus, in extreme cases of back pain,

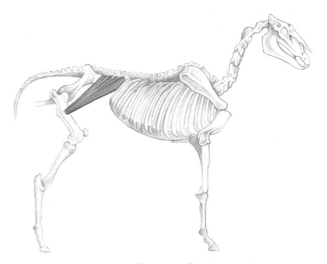

ILLUSTRATION 5A: Psoas in Quadrupeds

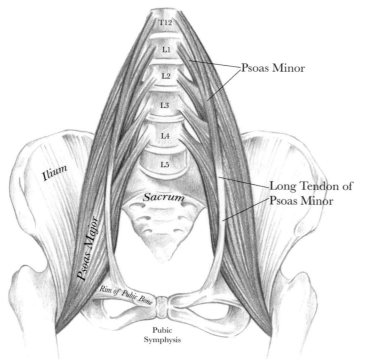

ILLUSTRATION 4: Psoas Minor

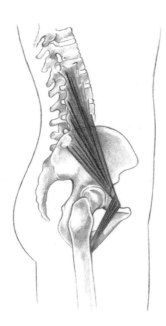

ILLUSTRATION 5B: Psoas in Biped

many people are reduced to crawling on all-fours, a position that takes pressure off of a contracted psoas. As you'll read in the *Red Flags* side bar (page 23), when the psoas is chronically tight, it most commonly pulls the lower back and pelvis into anterior rotation (hyperlordosis), and this is accentuated when the legs are straight. This is one reason many people find it uncomfortable to lie on their back with the legs straight and intuitively know to bend their knees to alleviate discomfort. Tightness in the psoas also can result in posterior rotation of the pelvis and flexion of the lower back (tucking the tail under and flattening the lumbar curvature), and this also can cause considerable discomfort in standing and lying down, as well as in movement (this paradoxical effect will be explained shortly). We'll make good use of this knowledge in Chapter Three when we explore several variations of a Constructive Rest Position as a go-to method for relaxing, releasing, and balancing the psoas.

Understanding how the psoas might contribute to both spinal flexion *and* extension involves a little conceptual leap. If you consider the psoas as six separate muscle bundles, each with its own unique pull and influence on the spine, we get a much better sense of how it actually functions. A muscle bundle of fibers extends sequentially from the 12th thoracic vertebra and each of the lumbar vertebrae to attach to the lesser trochanter of the femur (Illustration 3).[5] Each of the muscle bundles of the psoas has a different vector of force on the skeletal structure, and the sequencing of the attachments suggests that the upper and lower fibers of the psoas serve different functions. Tom Myers, author of *Anatomy Trains*, suggests that contraction of the upper fibers primarily contributes to spinal flexion and posterior rotation of the pelvis, and contraction of the lower fibers contributes to extension of the lumbar spine and anterior rotation of the pelvis (Illustrations 6A and 6B).[6,7] In a balanced psoas, these two actions potentially cancel each other out, with the spine being neither pulled into flexion nor extension but supported in a *neutral* lumbar curvature.

Let's pause here for a moment to anchor the concept of "neutral" spinal curves. Despite the common postural dictate to "stand up straight," the spinal column is not a straight rod, but it is designed to be sensuously curved. Spinal

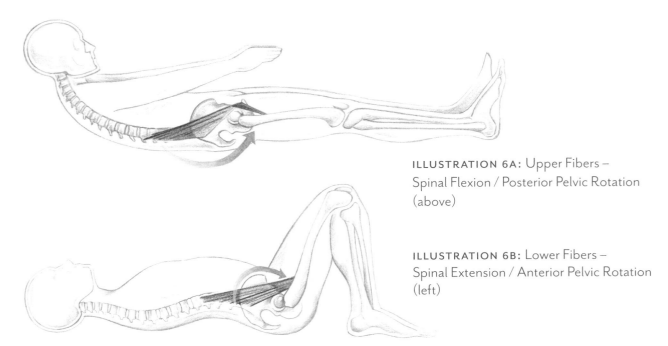

ILLUSTRATION 6A: Upper Fibers – Spinal Flexion / Posterior Pelvic Rotation (above)

ILLUSTRATION 6B: Lower Fibers – Spinal Extension / Anterior Pelvic Rotation (left)

curvatures not only increase shock absorption but also provide a central axis through which gravity must fall straight and true. The natural indentation of the lumbar curvature stacks the sturdy bodies of the vertebrae underneath the substantial weight of the structures above. Similarly, the natural indentation of the cervical vertebrae of the neck stacks these bones under the weight of the head. Neutral spinal curves occur when the cervical, thoracic, and lumbar curves are balanced over a stable pelvis so that the spinal vertebrae have maximum space between them (Illustration 7).

When the lumbar curve becomes too flat or is even reversed, this is called *hypolordosis*. When the lumbar curve becomes too accentuated, this is called *hyperlordosis*. The lumbar vertebrae can be pulled forward or back of an optimal curvature through an imbalance in the psoas. If the upper fibers of the psoas are too tight, they may pull the lumbar spine into flexion. If the lower fibers are too tight, they may pull the spine into extension. Other muscular imbalances, such as tight ham-

strings pulling on the sitting bones, can cause a posterior tilt of the pelvis. Thus, tight hamstrings can lead indirectly to a flattening of the lumbar curve. Inadequate support from weak abdominal muscles can cause an anterior tilt of the pelvis, contributing to an accentuation of the lumbar curve. Both hypo- and hyperlordosis can be congenital or can be caused by spinal degeneration. Regardless of the cause, a lumbar spine that has lost its neutral curvature also has lost its ability to channel the force of gravity and effectively absorb weight coming through the structure. We'll return to these concepts when we discuss how maintaining a neutral lumbar curvature affects core stability and movement.

Current research findings seem to indicate that not only do the upper and lower fibers have different functions but the superficial and deep fibers also have different roles. Although not all researchers are in agreement, the upper and deeper muscle bundles appear to function primarily as postural muscles providing spinal

✣ Finding a Neutral Pelvic Position

Stand with your feet hip-width apart and place your fingers on the creases of your groin just underneath your hip bones. Tuck your tail under and flatten your lower back (hypolordosis) and notice that the tissue under your fingers has become hard and sinewy. Now tip your pelvis forward so that the lumbar curve is accentuated (hyperlordosis) and notice that the tissue under your fingers has become like an over-soft mattress. Experiment by tipping the pelvis forward and back, alternating between the too-tight, too-soft sensations

under your fingers. Now make the movements smaller until you find a neutral pelvic position. In neutral, you should feel a "springy" sensation under your fingers. You are now standing with the pelvis centered over the legs. The weight of the upper body is now being supported by the bones of the pelvis, thighs, and lower legs. Trace your hands along the lumbar spine to feel the natural inward curve when you are in a neutral position. Take a few moments to let the rest of your body adjust and relax into this new postural awareness. ✣

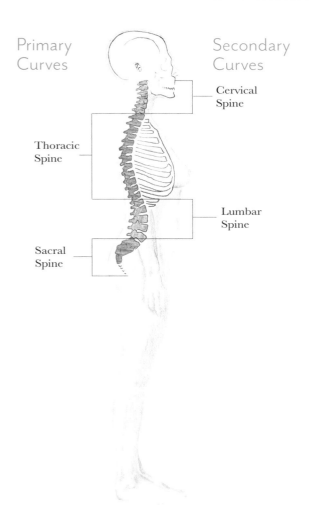

Primary
Curves

Secondary
Curves

Cervical
Spine

Thoracic
Spine

Lumbar
Spine

Sacral
Spine

ILLUSTRATION 7: Spinal Curves

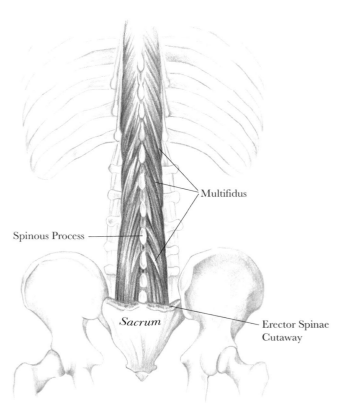

Multifidus

Spinous Process

Sacrum

Erector Spinae
Cutaway

ILLUSTRATION 8A: Multifidus

stability. The lower and more superficial muscle bundles are associated more strongly with movement such as flexing the hip.

Although we will explore other essential core muscles in Chapter Seven (pages 105–130), it is valuable to note that the way muscle bundles of the psoas relay up the spine share many characteristics with one of the other primary stabilizers of the spine—the *multifidus* (Illustration 8A). Both are the deepest muscles attached to the spine; the multifidus is on the back of the spine (posteriorly), whereas the psoas attaches to the side and front (laterally and anteriorly), of the vertebral bodies. This placement close to the central axis indicates their importance as postural muscles in maintain-

ing the verticality of the axis. Both muscle groups are arranged in overlapping bundles that permit individual activation of muscles between two spinal vertebrae as well as sequencing of movement and force over a greater length of the spine (Illustration 8B). Both muscles have a superficial and deep layer; the deep layers of multifidus connect to the transverse abdominis (the most interior of the four layers of the abdominal muscles), which is also a key stabilizer of the spine. The deep layers of the psoas connect to all the other core muscles. Both muscles suffer almost immediate atrophy as a result of spinal dysfunction, and research has shown that both muscles atrophy at the level of a prolapsed disk. Finally, both muscles will increase in cross-section with targeted core muscle rehabilitation, providing significant relief to individuals suffering pain and lumbar disability.

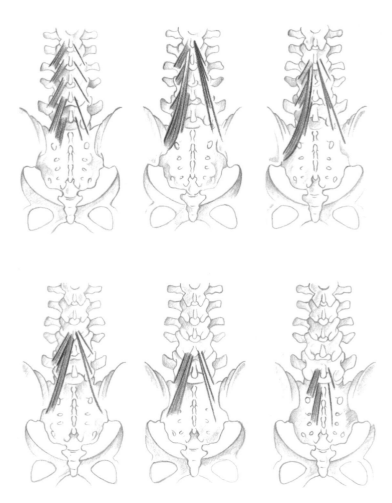

ILLUSTRATION 8B: Multifidus

The location of the psoas so close to the spine points to its prime importance as a core muscle. The large size of the psoas indicates its critical and far-reaching array of functions that include movement, stability, and force transmission. In traversing the body like a bridge, psoas major connects the spine to the legs. It is continually active when standing or sitting, as well as when the leg swings forward in walking.

The psoas often is referred to as the iliopsoas complex to acknowledge that psoas major shares its point of insertion with another muscle, the iliacus. The iliacus is a fan-shaped muscle that attaches from the inner surface of the ilia on each side of the pelvis and connects to the lesser trochanter via a common tendon with the psoas major (Illustration 9). It also attaches to both sacroiliac and lumbar ligaments. Although the psoas major connects the spine to the legs, the iliacus connects the pelvis to the legs. Working together with the psoas, this muscle gives force and endurance to hip flexion in movements such as kicking and running. Iliacus activity is minimal in standing but continuous in walking.

Key Concepts

▸ The iliopsoas is a structural bridge connecting the spine, the pelvis, and the legs.

▸ The psoas has multiple points of attachment, creating different vectors of force that work to either stabilize or move the spine, pelvis, and legs.

▸ The primary function of the psoas is to stabilize the spine. ❋

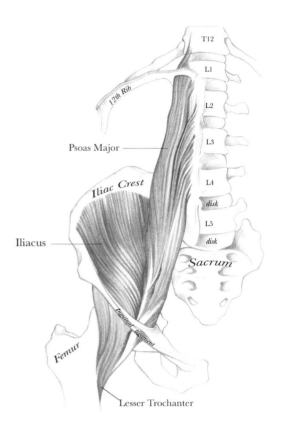

ILLUSTRATION 9: Iliacus

MOVEMENT FUNCTION OF THE PSOAS

If you were to attend an anatomy lecture more than twenty years ago, the section on the psoas would have been notably brief, declaring it to be a primary flexor of the hip in relation to the trunk, or a flexor of the trunk in relation to the hip. Or put more simply, the psoas can act as a pulley to draw the thighs in toward the abdomen or it can draw the abdomen and trunk toward the thighs. It was viewed as the primary muscle responsible for walking, and although elements of this are true, more recent research has challenged these basic assumptions. In fact, some researchers have disputed any movement of the spine or hip as the primary role of the psoas and instead have suggested stability as its primary function. Certainly when viewed in cross-section, it is visibly apparent that the psoas acts as an industrial-strength column of support girding each side of the lumbar spine (Illustration 10). Anatomically, the presence of so many other muscles that can accomplish the movements traditionally ascribed to the psoas lends itself to this argument. It is more likely that the psoas participates with other muscles

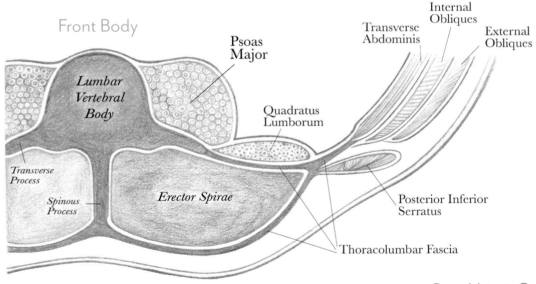

ILLUSTRATION 10: Psoas Major in Cross-Section

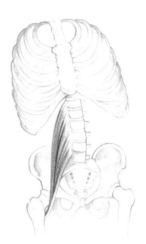

Unilateral Tightness of the Psoas

ILLUSTRATION 11A: Tightness of the psoas on one side of the body can draw the rib cage downward, and pull the lumbar spine off-center. This is a primary stage of compensation.

synergistically to accomplish movements. It could be hypothesized that as the deepest core muscle, the psoas is meant to initiate movement that other muscles then amplify and direct.

Paradoxically, although research supports the view that the psoas muscle is not a primary mover of the spine, when it is chronically contracted, it has the capacity to distort and misalign the spine and pelvis and to perpetuate that misalignment until it is released with proper treatment. This is especially true with one-sided (unilateral) tightness of the psoas (Illustration 11A).

Initially, unilateral tightness of the psoas can manifest as a shortening of the waist and lowering of the rib cage toward the side that is under tension, but secondary compensations almost inevitably follow, making both diagnosis and treatment tricky. Your eyes are always attempting to right themselves to the horizon (known as the Head Righting Reflex), and this eventually may lead to other secondary compensations such as scoliosis (lateral deviation of the spine), hip hiking (the femur or pelvis being raised), sacroiliac dysfunction, and inflammation of the lumbar fac-

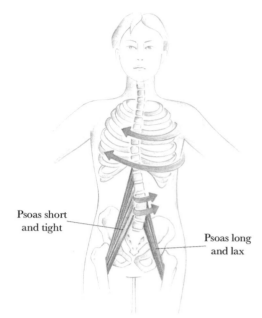

Psoas short
and tight

Psoas long
and lax

Secondary Compensations of Unilateral Psoas Tightness

ILLUSTRATION 11B: Secondary compensations can include, but are not limited to, hip hiking, rotation of the rib cage, rotation of the lumbar vertebrae, and sacroiliac dysfunction.

ets caused by compression and rotation of these vertebrae (Illustration 11B).

Unilateral contraction of the psoas almost always involves its neighbor, and sometimes partner in crime, quadratus lumborum (or QL as it is commonly known), which is also part of the posterior abdominal wall. QL originates from the posterior crest of the ilium and inserts onto the 12th rib and the transverse processes of the 1st–4th lumbar vertebrae (Illustration 12A). Its fibers run vertically and obliquely. Quadratus lumborum has three layers: a deep, middle, and superficial layer (Illustration 12B).

A pattern emerges here, in which it appears that the superficial portion of layered muscles like QL, multifidus, and the psoas is associated with movement, and the deeper portion is associated with stability. When the pelvis is fixed, contraction of quadratus lumborum on one side causes

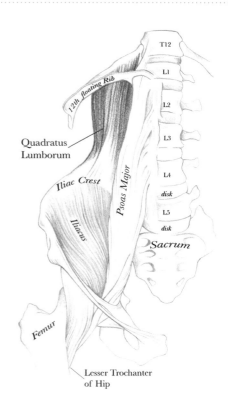

ILLUSTRATION 12A: Quadratus Lumborum

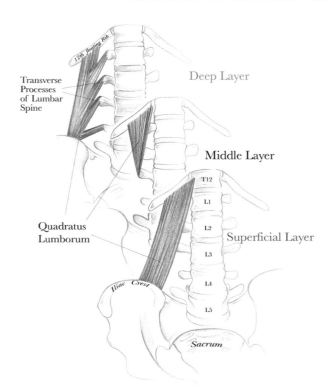

ILLUSTRATION 12B: The Three Layers of Quadratus Lumborum

side bending of the lumbar spine and rib cage. When the ribs and spine are fixed, it can raise the pelvis on one side. Thus, QL has the capacity to trigger imbalance in the psoas and vice versa. Inequities between the left and right QL can cause lateral flexion and rotation in the lumbar spine and hip hiking (Illustration 12C).

Research suggests that the way in which the psoas works also depends on the degree of flexion at the hip joint.[8] As the hip bone flexes more deeply, such as when you draw one leg into a high marching position, the psoas may become less of a spinal support and more of a hip flexor. In fact, the psoas, together with the iliacus, is the only muscle that can flex the hip bone more than 90 degrees in a standing position.

Dr. Nikolai Bogduk, who has been researching the anatomical basis of various spinal syndromes for forty years, and is a professor of Pain Medicine at the University of Newcastle, Australia, also has concluded from his studies that the main function

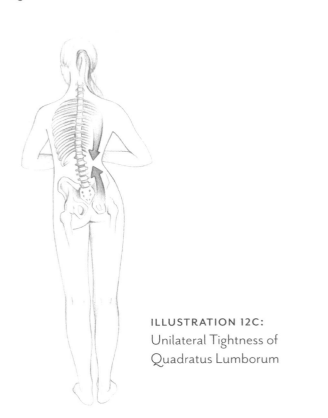

ILLUSTRATION 12C:
Unilateral Tightness of Quadratus Lumborum

of the psoas is to stabilize the lumbar spine through the mechanism of axial compression. Axial compression occurs when the psoas and other deep core muscles contract, causing an increase in the pressure in the abdomen. As a result, the disks become slightly compressed, creating a stiffening of the lumbar spine.[9] This prepares the spine for increased weight bearing, such as when you want to safely lift a heavy parcel. Think of axial compression as an internal scaffolding that stabilizes the lumbar vertebrae and the disks.

The psoas also influences the hip, helping to stabilize the head of the femur. Although the anatomical community disagrees about whether external rotation is also an action of the psoas, clinical experience supports this role. If you consider the way in which the lower fibers of the psoas and iliacus wrap medially to insert to the inside of the femur, this suggests that under tension, they contribute to the external rotation of the hip. If you are seated in a chair, you can mimic the external action of the psoas by taking hold of the inner seam of your pant leg and lifting up: if the leg is completely passive like that of a puppet, you'll find that the leg moves into slight external rotation. In our practice as Yoga teachers, we have observed that students who have difficulty keeping their thighs in a parallel position while lying on the floor with bent knees, often have very tight or incompetent psoas muscles (together with weak inner thigh muscles). This is the reason we may instruct you in many of the exercises that follow, to slightly *internally rotate* the thigh. This action can stabilize the insertion of the psoas and thus create a more effective release.

The conflicting schools of thought regarding psoas function and movement may reflect different intentions of researchers and clinicians. The ongoing disagreement in the research community (and between researchers and somatic practitioners) shows little sign of resolution, as information is being updated constantly by new research. The position taken in this book reflects the research that makes the most sense to us given our experience in translating that knowledge into effective practices for our students. Researchers often pursue a narrow research focus with objective criteria (often with the use of cadavers rather than living subjects), whereas practitioners tend to be more interested in functional effects, such as changes in alignment and posture, increased range of motion, improved strength, and greater coordination of movement. Somatic practitioners also recognize more subjective changes, such as greater ease in breathing or a felt sense of grounded stability. These experiences are difficult to quantify, but more subjective changes, such as ease in upright posture, fluency in walking, or improved sense of balance, will be of significance to anyone who wishes to move freely and without pain.

We also note a marked chasm between clinicians who have had extensive theoretical training but who themselves may have poor movement function, and somatic practitioners, such as those who teach Feldenkrais, Hanna Somatics, and the Alexander method and well-trained Yoga teachers who have spent decades developing a refined awareness of body movement. If someone does not have an embodied understanding of how to be functionally integrated in movement, it is unlikely that person would be able to teach others to move well. Many of the students who have come to us with long histories of back pain that have not been resolved through clinical intervention, often have been shown movements that are so grossly executed that their practice only serves to perpetuate compression, pain, and further injury. Additionally, helping our students and clients to develop a more refined awareness of their bodies takes time, patience, and consistent practice over several weeks and months. Structural imbalance is usually the result of decades of poor posture and poor movement habits. Learning new ways of moving and both releasing and strengthening the structure so that it is "self-supporting" cannot be acquired through passive manual therapy alone but only may be achieved through the active participation of a person motivated to practice self-care.

What is true about the nature and function of the psoas may vary from person to person as this vital muscle is sensed, felt, and moved in the laboratory of the body. Ultimately, the proof is in the pudding—being able to center your body and move with stability will make an incredible difference not only in all your everyday activities but also in your deeper sense of being mentally and emotionally balanced.

☀ Key Concepts

▸ An unbalanced psoas can pull the pelvis off-center and distort the neutral spinal curvatures.

▸ When the psoas co-contracts with other core muscles, the action of axial compression stabilizes the spine.

▸ Long and strong psoas muscles support ease in spinal and hip movement. ❋

❖ Red Flags

What are some of the signs that indicate that the psoas may be the culprit in contributing to spinal discomfort, pain, or movement restriction? Do you notice any of these symptoms?

Pain: You suffer from groin, lower or mid-back pain, sacroiliac discomfort, or sciatica, and the symptoms are significantly lessened after you practice a psoas release movement, especially one using a Muscle Release Ball (MR Ball).

Standing: You are able to bring your pelvis into a neutral position if you bend your knees, but as soon as you straighten the legs, the pelvis moves into an anterior tilt (hyperlordosis) or posterior tilt (hypolordosis). You have lost the ability to flex or extend the femur in the hip socket without altering the position of the pelvis.

Sitting: You feel a painful "catch" in your groin when standing up from prolonged sitting, particularly when your legs have been crossed. It may take you a while to ease up to a vertical position. You may have pain in your lower back when sitting or when transitioning from sitting to standing.

Lying Down: While lying on your back you feel the need to keep your knees bent. Straightening your legs causes immediate tension and discomfort in the lower back or sacroiliac joints.

Back Bending: When bending backward you feel compression or pain in your lower back, especially at the juncture between L5 and S1 (where the lower back and sacrum meet) or at the juncture between T12 and L1 (where the rib cage ends and the lower back begins). You may find it difficult to achieve full extension in your groins in back bends.

One-Sided Lower Back Tension or Pain: You notice persistent tension or pain on one side of your lower or mid-back. This unilateral discomfort may increase with extension (back bending). A unilateral pull of the psoas and its partner in crime, QL, may be the source of this discomfort. If symptoms and pain caused by sacroiliac or sciatic issues are lessened significantly after you practice psoas release movements (especially practices utilizing the MR Ball), these muscles are probably the culprits.

Forward Bending: You initiate forward bending by "see-sawing" at the base of the rib cage or the lumbosacral junction, rather than hinging at the hips. You may struggle to pause in a tabletop position or in a standing forward bend, or you may tend to "fall" into standing forward bends rather than moving with a controlled descent.

Hip Flexion: When you bring the knee into the chest you feel pinching or pain in the groin.

External Rotation: Your knees and legs turn outward when you lie down in Constructive Rest Position or the preparation for a Bridge Pose (*Setu Bandhasana*; see page 125). When you try to maintain your thighs in a parallel position, the adductors (inner thigh muscles) tire and may even begin to tremble. Some-

times the legs reflexively fall outward despite your best efforts. Because the psoas contributes to external rotation of the hip, a short and tight psoas can cause these symptoms.

Bridging of the Rib Cage: Your lower ribs poke forward when you bring your arms over your head. Remember that the psoas attaches at the juncture between the rib cage and the lumbar spine. If it is tight, you'll be unable to keep your rib cage in a neutral position with the arms overhead.

Other Musculoskeletal Symptoms: Psoas dysfunction can contribute to chronic hip flexion, disk protrusion, an apparent short leg, over development of anterior thigh muscles (quads), restricted movement of the hip socket, and forward head posture.

Other causative factors may contribute to all of these red flags. If in doubt, consider seeing your health-care practitioner to obtain proper diagnosis and treatment. In particular, pain that is not relieved by any change of position is a serious warning signal and should be cause to immediately see a medical professional. ❖

COHESION AND CORE INITIATION OF MOVEMENT

Cohesion in movement is a result of all the body parts working in collective agreement to accomplish a given task. When each part of the body makes its rightful contribution of effort, the whole body moves in unity. You could think of your psoas as being the muscle that stands in the center of the body and conducts and orchestrates this cohesiveness.

Two seemingly opposing forces create the qual-

ity of cohesion. Although the psoas muscles can *shorten and contract* when flexing or extending the spine and hip, they also can *lengthen and contract*. An eccentric muscle contraction is a type of muscle activation in which the muscle *lengthens* and *narrows* as it contracts, moving the two ends farther apart, which results in extension of a joint. Eccentric contractions are common to many sports and activities for which you need controlled or resisted

❖ Body Stories: Standing Up Straight for the First Time

When Alevia attended a "Moving from the Core" intensive workshop, she hoped to find some answers to her long-standing hyper-lordotic back. When upright, she described her experience as having a "butt that is one foot behind me and a stomach that is one foot in front of me." The simple act of standing upright felt like a struggle as she battled to bring her tipped-forward pelvis into some semblance of neutral. After each psoas exercise, our study group would observe the change in Alevia's supine position and later in her standing posture. By the end of the day, she had radically reduced the gapping hollow between her lumbar spine and the floor. Standing up, she shared that it felt for the first time like she truly had stood up straight. ❖

types of movement, for instance, walking down stairs, lowering a heavy parcel onto the floor, running downhill, or slowly lowering the pelvis back onto the floor as in a Yoga posture, such as Bridge Pose (see page 125). Learning how to consciously elongate the psoas while it works leads to a long and strong lower back. For example, in a standing forward bend, eccentric contraction of the psoas muscle supports the spine in a controlled descent toward the floor. Eccentric activation of muscles is associated with greater muscle strengthening than concentric muscle activation.

In concentric muscle contraction the muscle *shortens* and *thickens* as the two ends move closer together, creating increased tension in the muscle and flexing the joint. This type of contraction takes place when lifting a heavy parcel from the floor or swinging the leg forward to take a step (one of the functions of the psoas). We know from our work as teachers how powerful ideokinetic imagery works on a neurological level: when students can see a muscle in their mind's eye, this immediately increases electrical impulse to that structure. What you can see you can activate, what you can engage you can use. Being able to consciously lengthen or shorten the psoas can

bring immediate gains in strength and cohesiveness when you move.

No muscle, however, works in isolation. The ability of the psoas to support the spine vitally depends on the coordinated engagement of the muscles of the abdomen and other muscles of the back. Although the abdominal muscles primarily offer more superficial frontal support to the body, the multifidus, psoas, and QL act more like guy-wires relaying up the back. Guy-wires frequently are used in construction to anchor cell towers, and on sail boats, acting as tensioned cables to stabilize a freestanding structure such as a mast. In the garden, guy-wires attached to the trunk of a bent tree can straighten the tree over time (Illustration 13). If you imagine the body as a sandwich, the abdominal muscles form the front layer, the psoas and QL are the filling, and the multifidus is the back layer. Both the front and back layers are important for strength and endurance but are best used as auxiliary reinforcement once the psoas is engaged. We'll expand on the role of these other core muscles and their contribution to body stability in Chapter Seven (pages 105–130).

Many of our students quickly discover that they chronically overuse their back and abdomi-

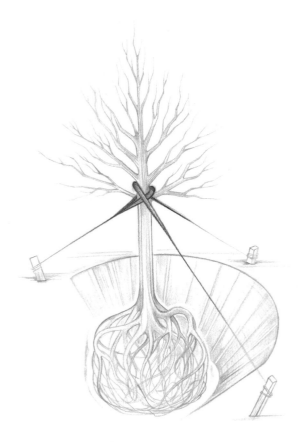

ILLUSTRATION 13: The fibers of the psoas act like guy-wires to stabilize and balance the spine.

nal muscles because of insufficient balance and support from the more central psoas. Because the more superficial abdominal muscles and quadriceps (*rectus femoris*) can replicate the action of the psoas but with far greater effort, we call these muscles the *superficial duplicators*. People who

move primarily from these superficial duplicators move in an effortful, uncoordinated way, often most apparent in walking. The legs may appear to have no functional relationship to the core of the body, moving in a puppet-like fashion. In her ground-breaking work *Rolfing: The Integration of Human Structures*, Ida Rolf states that "the legs do not originate movement in the walk of a balanced body: the legs support and follow. Movement is initiated in the trunk and transmitted to the legs through the medium of the psoas."[10]

When the psoas is accessed with awareness and is engaged appropriately, movement emanates from the center of the body and is ultimately more integrated and graceful. Imagining the legs beginning from the origin of the psoas at the level of the 12th thoracic vertebra is an effective way of feeling how this relay occurs from the core all the way down to the feet.

❀ Key Concepts

▸ Core movement is initiated from the psoas with the other core muscles taking a supporting role.

▸ The superficial duplicators (the quadriceps and external abdominal muscles) can replicate the action of the psoas but with far greater effort.

▸ Learning to engage the psoas as the primary mover allows more superficial muscles to relax and release. ❀

SPINAL STABILITY AND UPRIGHT POSTURE

Mabel Todd, the grandmother of movement therapy, regarded the psoas as the most important muscle in determining upright posture.[11] Simply put, the psoas determines the position of the pelvis and the position of the pelvis determines the position of the spine. Paradoxically, the psoas is not only the most important muscle in determin-

ing erect posture but also the muscle that holds and reinforces compensatory misalignments that distort the spine.

The degree of engagement of the psoas determines whether a person is able to "stand in their bones" with a clear sequencing of force from the upper to the lower body (Illustration 14A). When

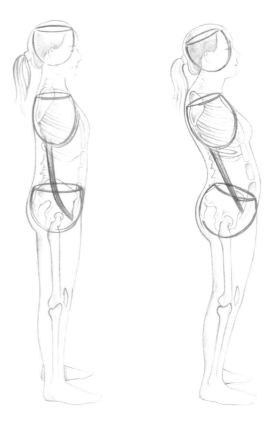

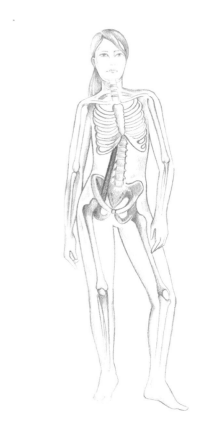

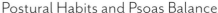

Postural Habits and Psoas Balance

ILLUSTRATION 14C

ILLUSTRATION 14A (left image): Good postural habits transfer weight load through the bones of the skeleton. In this scenario the psoas muscles become long and strong.

ILLUSTRATION 14B (right image): Poor postural habits shift weight load to the joints, ligaments, tendons, and internal organs. In this scenario the psoas muscles become shortened and weak.

the body parts have no collective agreement about their relationship to ground, gravity, and space, or to each other, the skeletal structure no longer acts as the primary support of weight. When this occurs, weight is instead born through the muscles, tendons, ligaments, and the internal organs (Illustration 14B). A casual glance at any social gathering will reveal how commonly people stand by shifting the hips to one side, collapsing into joints and leaning against ligaments, rather than standing balanced between their two feet

(Illustration 14C). This asymmetrical shift in the structure may become more permanent through innocent practices, such as habitually carrying a child on one hip (Illustration 14D). Increasingly, we are seeing preadolescent students with pronounced kyphosis (increased thoracic curvatures) and problems with both neck and lower back through being chronically flexed over a computer, laptop, game console, or cell phone (Illustration 14E). All these practices create imbalances in the core psoas muscles. Bones, not soft tissues, are designed to bear weight and transfer load, so when skeletal misalignment displaces load onto the psoas muscle, it obliges by becoming hard and rigid like bone. Unfortunately, when this occurs, a vicious cycle is set in place, with the chronic tightness perpetuating the postural imbalance, and the postural imbalance perpetuating a tight, unyielding psoas.

Balanced between stability and flexibility, an

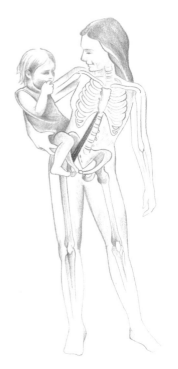

ILLUSTRATION 14D

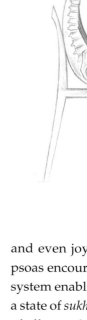

ILLUSTRATION 14E

engaged psoas significantly decreases the amount of effort required to stand upright by allowing the body to rely on the skeleton for support and by enabling the muscles to organize themselves around an open and resilient core. A basic concept in many movement disciplines is *what is lacking below will be compensated for higher up*. When the legs, pelvis, and lower back fail to do their job of supporting the body's weight, structures higher up in the body accumulate tension. When foundational support is sufficient in the lower body, the jaw, neck, and shoulders relax and release. Instead of using superficial muscular effort to stay upright, psoas engagement encourages trust in the skeletal system so that the muscles can stream along the bones as auxiliary support.

In Patanjali's Yoga Sutra II:46, asana or posture is defined as *Sthira sukham asanam*. *Sthira* has been translated variously to mean "steady, alert, stable, and strong." *Sukha* is translated as a "good or pleasant space" and is the consort and counterbalance of *sthira*, offering comfort, relaxation, ease,

and even joy. Thus, one could say that a happy psoas encourages trust in the *sthira* of the skeletal system enabling the muscular system to relax into a state of *sukha*. This balance between the dualities of effort and relaxation lie at the heart of comfortable and sustainable posture and movement.

✺ *Key Concepts*

▸ Bones not muscles are designed to carry weight.

▸ Poor postural habits contribute to chronic psoas imbalance.

▸ A centered pelvis is the key to good posture. ✺

THE PSOAS AND SACROILIAC STABILITY

The sacroiliac (SI) joint is the meeting place between the large triangular sacral bone and the two ilia of the pelvis (Illustration 15A). The joint is tacked together by a veritable fortress of liga-

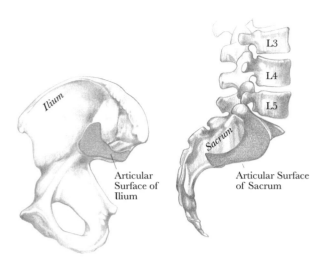

ILLUSTRATION 15A: Sacroiliac Joint Articulations

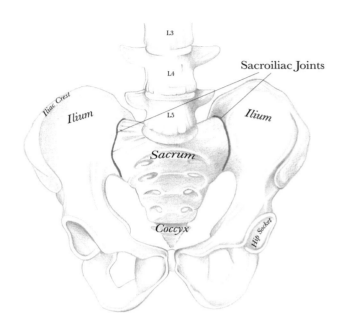

ILLUSTRATION 15C: Sacroiliac Joints

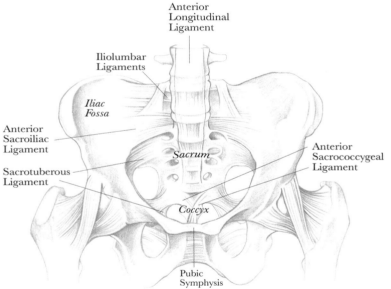

ILLUSTRATION 15B: Sacroiliac Ligaments Anterior

a stable SI joint to be transmitted without causing damage. We will elaborate in Chapter Seven on other essential core muscles, but for now, it's helpful to know that research confirms that the psoas muscles contribute to the healthy snug fit of the SI joint.[12] Too much shortening of the psoas, however, can cause excessive compression through these joints, causing pain and restricted movement.

Understanding this fit of the SI joint is significant because we are seeing a worldwide epidemic of SI instability in Yoga practitioners who have sacrificed stability and strength in their bodies in ambitious pursuit of extreme pretzel-like poses. SI hypermobility is often the result of forcing the femur beyond a healthy range of motion such that it becomes a lever to pry the SI joints apart. Once the ligaments of the SI joint have been overstretched through this extreme leveraging, the resulting hypermobility of the joint can be corrected only through strengthening regional

mentous tissue, yet has almost no direct muscular support (Illustration 15B). The SI joint acts as the central hub of the skeletal structure, coordinating transmission of force into and out of the center of the body (Illustration 15C). All of the force coming up from the ground to the pelvis or down through the spine to the pelvis must be mediated through core muscles. Regional core muscles sometimes are referred to as "local stabilizers," the deep core muscles that attach to the vertebrae and are capable of sustained contraction. Their primary function is to provide stability between the segments of the spine. Significantly, students who have come to us with long-standing misalignment and discomfort of the SI joint often report that many of the psoas releases have immediately reduced their SI pain. Considering how much influence the iliopsoas complex can have on the position of the pelvis, any realignment of the pelvic bones into better balance supports the optimal function of the sacroiliac joint. And like so many of the circular relationships we have seen between anatomical structures, optimal SI function also supports optimal lower back and hip function.

❀ Key Concepts

▸ A balanced psoas can help to release a restricted SI joint.

▸ Overstretching the SI ligaments can cause SI instability.

▸ Strengthening regional core muscles can stabilize the SI joint. ❀

FASCIA AND THE PSOAS

Traditionally, fascia has been used as a medical term applying to specific sheets of biological fabric in the body, such as the plantar fascia (on the bottom of the foot) or the thoracolumbar fascia (on either side of the lower back). Increasingly, somatic practitioners such as Thomas Myers and other researchers are challenging this limited definition of fascia. Their work suggests that fascia is a three-dimensional fibrous web of protein, and it is one continuous anatomical network throughout the body. Viewed from this perspective, fascia is a regulatory system for the biomechanics of the body. This broader definition of fascia as "all the collagenous-based soft tissue of the body" includes all the tissues classically defined as fascia plus other tissues, such as tendons and ligaments, as well as the fascia in and around the muscles, nerves, and organs.

The psoas has intimate fascial connections to many structures, including the diaphragm, the pelvic floor, QL, multifidus, and the anterior spinal ligament (the long band of "duct tape" that stabilizes the front of the spine). Through its relationship to the diaphragm, the psoas is connected to the cardiovascular system, the kidneys, and the deep fascia of the front of the neck. Although the connection between the psoas and legs clearly is defined by the arrangement of muscles, the relationship between the psoas and arms is less obvious because the link is through the fascia. The fascia of three major shoulder muscles—the trapezius, latissimus dorsi, and pectoralis major—forms a muscular plane through the deep fascia that attaches to the midline.[13] The Celestial Design Committee clearly wanted to connect the upper limbs (arms) to the lower limbs (legs) through the nexus of a midpoint. Why are these pervasive fascial connections between the psoas and other structures significant? Clinical research has determined that fascia contains *six times more sensory nerve endings than muscle.*[14] This has exciting implications for the psoas muscle as a sensory organ.[15]

Research has shown that often a muscular or motor problem is primarily a sensory problem and that training sensory awareness gives the brain the stimulus it needs to improve movement.[16] The extensive fascial component and sensory innervation of the large psoas muscle may contribute to maintenance of upright posture by sensing and registering changes in terrain, load, position, and stress, relaying this information to the central nervous system and implementing any adjustments or compensations necessary to maintain the eyes level with the horizon (known as the Head Righting Reflex). When the Head Righting Reflex is activated by uneven terrain or a distortion somewhere in the musculoskeletal structure, it is conceivable that the psoas bears some of the burden of attempting to level the eyes with the horizon by contracting or inhibiting whatever muscle bundles will accomplish this task. With so many receptors in its pervasive fascia and with its numerous muscle bundles angled at different vectors, the psoas would be well suited for the job.

Consider how the sensory function of the psoas may be compromised when it is chronically tight or underutilized. If the proprioceptors in the muscle and fascia of the psoas are acting as an internal navigational system, any imbalance in the psoas potentially could cause inefficient and unbalanced weight transfer to the SI joints, hips, knees, and ankles, much like a navigational system that has gone awry, sending you on wild detours through side streets rather than taking the most efficient route. This inefficient routing of force through the body can cause excessive and uneven loading into joints such as the knee, leading to deterioration of the joint surfaces and premature degeneration.

When we translate these anatomical insights into movement, it's helpful to incorporate one more fascinating quality of fascia: *viscoelasticity*. As Yoga teacher and researcher Clare Raffety points out, "while the fascial system connects, separates, transmits forces, and acts as a key communication pathway . . . it is also a viscous system, which can exhibit more liquid or more crystalline qualities in different situations and internal environment."[17] The fascia, like your ligaments and tendons, has the ability to resist deformation when force or stress is applied. You can observe this phenomenon when trying to pull apart warm toffee. Viscoelasticity becomes important when you start to use visual imagery while lengthening or shortening the psoas muscle. Viscoelasticity in the fascial tissue causes a resistance or "pull back" that contributes to the quality of cohesion when the psoas is activated or lengthened. This interplay of dynamic tension contributes to greater stability within the muscle fibers and reduces potential injury, especially to the spine.

Although a more thorough discussion of fascia is outside the scope of this book, the traditional view of muscles moving bones gradually is giving way to a new paradigm that explains our form, relationship to gravity, alignment, and movement in terms of a unified tensional network formed by the entire fascia in the body. This unified network suspends the bones and transfers loads and forces in an omnidirectional way. This emerging paradigm may explain how we can balance gravity and the counterthrust of gravity in whatever position we take.

❋ Key Concepts

▶ Fascia is the continuous biological fabric of the body that both connects and separates structures.

▶ Fascia is highly innervated with sensory nerve receptors.

▶ The fascia in the psoas registers changes in the body's position and rights itself accordingly. ❋

THE PSOAS AND BREATHING

Although the thoracic diaphragm generally is considered to be the primary breathing muscle, its role as a core stabilizer increasingly has been acknowledged. We will more thoroughly explain

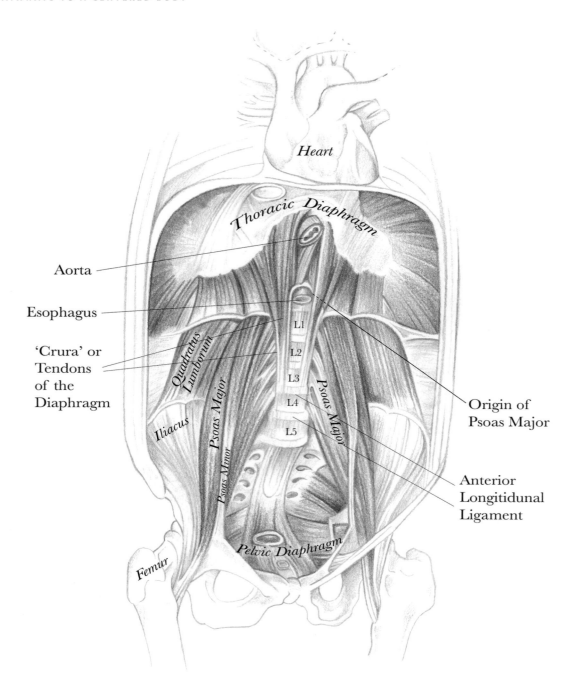

Heart

Thoracic Diaphragm

Aorta

Esophagus

'Crura' or
Tendons
of the
Diaphragm

L1

L2

L3

L4

L5

Quadratus
Lumborum

Psoas Major

Iliacus

Psoas Minor

Psoas Major

Origin of
Psoas Major

Anterior
Longitidunal
Ligament

Pelvic Diaphragm

Femur

The Diaphragm and the Psoas

ILLUSTRATION 16: The long tendons of the diaphragm interweave with fibers of the psoas major at its point of origin. The tendons of the diaphragm also interweave with the anterior longitudinal ligament (ALL), which runs like duct tape all the way down to the tail. As the diaphragm ascends and descends, the tendons pull on the ALL, conveying an oscillatory movement all the way down to the sacrum and tail.

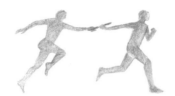

Psoas-Diaphragm Relay

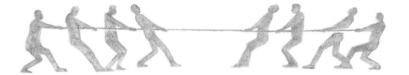

Psoas-Diaphragm Tug of War

ILLUSTRATION 17: Communication Between the Psoas and Diaphragm

the significance of the diaphragm as a core stabilizer in Chapter Seven. For now, understanding the anatomical relationship of the diaphragm to the psoas gives us clues as to why balancing the psoas can result in better breathing.

The attachments of the psoas and the thoracic diaphragm liberally overlap at their shared point of origin along the lumbar spine. If you recall, psoas major arises from the 12th thoracic to the 5th lumbar vertebrae. The double-domed diaphragm anchors itself to the lumbar spine via tendons called *crura*, which attach to the bodies of the 1st to the 3rd lumbar vertebrae. The muscle fibers of the psoas and diaphragm muscle interdigitate at their common attachments on these three lumbar vertebrae (Illustration 16). This interweaving of muscular fibers can act as a communication juncture between the two structures so that impulse is effectively relayed from the psoas to the diaphragm and vice versa, much like handing over a baton in a relay race. However, when either the psoas or diaphragm is bound with tension, the junction between the two structures can act more like a tug of war (Illustration 17).

A chronically tight psoas can inhibit the free movement of the diaphragm, and any loss of free-dom in the free rise and fall of the diaphragm can impair the function of the psoas. The psoas and diaphragm co-contract; when the psoas muscles are hypertonic (chronically contracted), the diaphragm follows suit, and its ability to descend on inhalation becomes compromised. Whenever the movement of a muscle is restricted to a small range of motion, its fascia becomes dense and hard. This hardening of the fascia can result in further movement inhibition—like trying to drive your car with the handbrake on. This can perpetuate a vicious cycle of contraction, restricted movement, and breathing dysfunction. The close connection between the psoas and respiratory diaphragm explains why breathing practices often relieve lower back pain.

A contracted psoas commonly results in a forward thrust of the rib cage, which puts pressure on both the front and back of the diaphragm. Conversely, contraction of other parts of the psoas muscle bundles can cause the spine to flex, rounding the back and compressing the front of the diaphragm. A contraction of the psoas on one side can rotate the rib cage to the opposite side, creating a torque through the diaphragm. Each of these misalignments will affect the action of breathing, often by restricting the abdominal and diaphragmatic breath capacity and encouraging upper chest breathing with its overuse of secondary respiratory muscles. Paradoxical breathing in particular (breathing movements in which the chest wall moves in on inspiration and out on expiration, in reverse of the normal movements) can thwart recovery of a dysfunctional psoas. Tension in the neighboring QL and multifidus muscles also will prevent freedom of the breath. Ironically, statically contracting the abdomen as is so commonly practiced to give the appearance of a flat tummy (code name, core fitness!), also can inhibit the full descent of the diaphragm. When the diaphragm cannot fully descend, this can trigger chest breathing—a way of breathing in which the secondary respiratory muscles high up in the chest, shoulders, and neck become the dominant, and inefficient, movers of the breath.

Although freedom of the movement of the diaphragm has immediate consequences for the process of breathing, full and easeful excursion of the diaphragm also acts to rhythmically massage the internal organs above and below the diaphragm. When both the diaphragm or psoas muscles do not function in a balanced way, the organs do not receive this massaging action, and their function can be affected adversely.

The deep structural interconnections between the diaphragm and the psoas muscles invite us to reconsider the paradigm of these central structures as separate muscles with discrete functions and open the way to view them as a continuous interrelated network.

✿ Key Concepts

▶ The psoas and diaphragm are connected intimately by overlapping attachments and fascia such that each has a significant effect on the health and function of the other.

▶ When the diaphragm contracts so does the psoas and vice versa.

▶ A tight psoas or diaphragm can cause misalignments in the pelvis, spine, and rib cage resulting in breath restriction.

▶ When the diaphragm and psoas muscles are balanced, the rhythmic action of breathing massages organs and improves their healthy functioning. ✾

THE PSOAS AND HEART HEALTH

Because of the heart's intimate connection to the diaphragm, any inhibition of its wave-like movements can have profound consequences for heart health. The heart lies right on top of the central tendinous portion of the diaphragm and is attached to the diaphragm by fascia (Illustration 18). Each time we breathe, the heart is massaged. As Dr. Andrew Thomas postulated in an extract from the *Journal of the International Yoga Therapists*, the fact that the heart is fascially bound to the diaphragm directly, and indirectly bound to the sternum and lower neck joints, would seem to be an arrangement intended to ensure manipulation by diaphragmatic action. Were this not so, it would have been a simple matter for the Celestial Design Committee to detach the heart from the diaphragm and anchor it instead to a rigid structure such as the sternum. Dr. Thomas writes:

The fascial connection is so widespread that it is clear that any diaphragmatic movement will cause heart migration and, it is reasonable to assume, cause changes in shape—a *sort of built in heart massage* [author's emphasis] . . . because the Vena

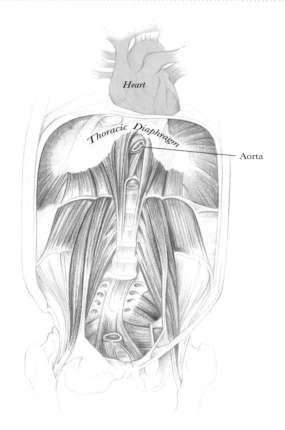

Heart

Thoracic Diaphragm

Aorta

ILLUSTRATION 18: The heart is bound by fascia to the diaphragm. Any inhibition of the full movement of breathing can, therefore, affect the healthy function of the heart.

Cava (the blood vessel that returns blood to the heart) pierces the diaphragm, the action described above causes the Vena Cava to be increased in size momentarily, which in turn reduces pipe blood pressure and allows an acceleration of blood flow back to the heart. The fully and correctly operating diaphragm is thus *a second heart*.[18]

A number of significant studies have shown a correlation between upper chest breathing (i.e.,

overuse of the secondary respiratory muscles and underuse of the thoracic diaphragm) and heart disease. In one sobering report, patients who already had experienced a heart attack were taught how to breathe diaphragmatically and to generalize this behavior into everyday activities. In doing so, they significantly reduced their chance of a second heart attack.[19] Another study showed that all 153 patients of a coronary unit breathed predominantly in their chests.[20]

If you recall the diaphragm's shared attachment with the psoas at the 1st–3rd lumbar vertebrae, and the interweaving of their fibers, tightness of the psoas directly inhibits the action of the diaphragm, and the resulting obstruction to breathing can affect the optimal function of the heart. So, it is not surprising that many of our students notice that after practicing psoas release exercises, they feel greater ease in the whole process of breathing. And what goes around comes around: this softening of the diaphragm and reactivation of its fibers as the primary mover of the breath serves to fluidly release the psoas.

❀ Key Concepts

▸ The heart sits right on top of the diaphragm and is massaged during breathing by its rhythmical up-and-down movements.

▸ When healthy movement of the diaphragm is restricted by tension in the psoas muscles, heart health can be affected.

▸ Releasing the psoas muscles can free the diaphragm and potentially improve heart function. ❀

THE PSOAS AND THE NERVOUS SYSTEM

As one of the leading somatic researchers of our time, Ida Rolf astutely has noted the way in which the solar plexus, a hub of nerves otherwise

know as the celiac plexus, lies approximately at the level where the psoas and diaphragm meet.[21] Nerves exiting the lumbar spine form the lumbar

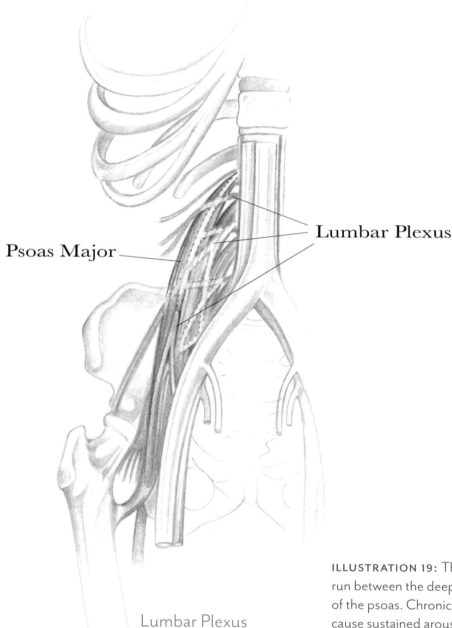

Psoas Major

Lumbar Plexus

Lumbar Plexus

ILLUSTRATION 19: The nerves of the solar plexus run between the deep and superficial fibers of the psoas. Chronic tension in the psoas can cause sustained arousal of the fight-or-flight reflex.

plexus, which is embedded in the surface of the psoas itself (Illustration 19). According to Rolf, any restriction of movement or excessive tension in the psoas could affect general metabolic functions as these are orchestrated by the autonomic nervous system.

The lumbar plexus of nerves is contained within the psoas *between the superficial and deep layers* and supplies innervation to some abdominal, pelvic, hip, and thigh muscles. The plexus, together with the large number of sensory neurons in psoas fascia, may be connected to the enteric nervous system, otherwise known as the abdominal brain. The sensing of "gut feelings" through the primitive abdominal brain may be registered by the psoas and an appropriate reaction mediated through the psoas. Long before the cerebral cortex even acknowledges a threat, the abdominal brain has registered its fear reaction with the psoas almost instantaneously contracting in defense. Even a mild response to fear, such as anxiety (i.e., "butterflies in the stomach"), can cause psoas and diaphragmatic contraction.

Because of its connections to the sympathetic nervous system, the psoas is the major muscle affected by the fight-or-flight reflex. Whenever a fear response is activated, the psoas readies the body to fight in defense, to escape by mobilizing the body into movement, or by freezing and playing dead in a protective fetal position. Our sophisticated prefrontal cortex can override this impulse to fight, take flight, or freeze, producing a "fake-it" response that can have us shaking in our boots while presenting an apparently calm demeanor. Our Paleolithic ancestors responded to danger through brisk and vigorous spikes of movement followed by periods of rest, dissipating stress chemicals from the body. Spinning our wheels while sitting at our desk chair can lead to skyrocketing levels of cortisol and other stress chemicals, which only perpetuate the stress response. Unfortunately, in modern times, our nervous system probably receives more stimulation in one day than our Paleolithic ancestors received in their entire lifetime, yet the hard wiring of the nervous system has changed little over millions of years. Being cut off in traffic, rushing to an appointment, or feeling intimidated by a colleague's comments, and other stressors can trigger this red-light response many times in the course of a day. Eventually, this can result in a chronic state of sympathetic arousal that can lead to adrenal exhaustion. Even after the source of our agitation is long gone, our bodies still may be flooded with stress chemicals such as cortisol.

The ongoing physical, mental, and emotional stress experienced by so many people in the twenty-first century can create a chronic contraction of the psoas. "Holding on" may become our modus operandi, rather than a more sustainable relaxed state of alertness and resiliency. Chronic tension in the psoas can cause persistent and sustained overactivation of the sympathetic nervous system. When you factor in additional tension caused by the average number of hours people spend in prolonged sitting positions, it's easy to recognize that an increase in sympathetic nervous system tone can contribute to a plethora of health problems.

Because of its intimate proximity to so many nerves, muscular contraction in the psoas can compress nerve fibers, affecting both somatic and autonomic nervous systems. Thus, a tight psoas can block or interfere with the sensory role of the psoas so that our perception of physical sensations, feelings, and emotions may be dulled causing us to lose touch with ourselves. Kinesthetic dystonia—or an inability to feel and make sense of what we feel—can result, leaving us without an internal navigational guidance system.

Kinesthesia is the sixth sense responsible for feeling. It is an interoceptive sensory perception—that is, it registers information about where the body is and how the body is, and it can be acquired only as we heighten our awareness of interior body sensation. Thus, kinesthesia is always an *inside job*; the person most capable of registering bodily sensation (and assigning meaning to those sensations) is the person living in that body. Conscious connection and release of the psoas can improve perception of body sensation as well as our ability to read our emotions.

For many clinicians working in the field of trauma relief, the psoas appears to be a repository for body memories and emotions, especially fear. Memories that may have been long buried can be stimulated by something as simple as a smell, a loud noise, or a face that looks familiar, triggering seemingly irrational behavior and reactive holding within the body. Any unconscious and persistent holding in the body causes a daily depletion of energy, energy that once liberated can be used toward better purposes. Gently releasing the psoas can result in a spontaneous welling of feelings often described as "coming out of nowhere," without a specific storyline attached to the experience. Nonetheless, these emotions may be experienced as an intense overflowing and release of feeling.

Mindfully accessing and consciously relaxing the psoas can moderate the balance between the sympathetic nervous system, which prepares the body and mind for alertness and action, and the parasympathetic nervous system, which regulates rest and restoration, including regulation of the body's unconscious actions, such as slowing the heart rate or increasing intestinal activity. Learning to soften and release your psoas also sets the stage for you to reset the nervous system (balancing sympathetic and parasympathetic function).

This increases your capacity to deal with stress, builds responsiveness rather than reactiveness, and cultivates resilience.

❀ Key Concepts

▸ Important nerves innervating the organs and legs are embedded in the psoas muscle.

▸ Chronic tightness in the psoas can trigger chronic stress responses.

▸ Releasing the psoas can support a healthy nervous system and increase the body's ability to relax and repair itself. ❀

❖ The Psoas, Vagal Tone, and Heart Rate Variability

The benefits of working with the psoas reflect good vagal tone and can be measured through heart rate variability. It is worth taking time to understand these concepts. The main nerve of the autonomic nervous system, the vagus nerve, innervates most of the organs with both a sympathetic and parasympathetic branch. Organ functions can be turned up or down according to what is necessary to maintain homeostasis. Vagal tone is a measurement of the state and level of activation of the vagus nerve and the autonomic nervous system. Good vagal tone is indicated by strong digestion, a low and robust pulse, stable moods, appropriate response to stressors, resiliency, and an ability to manage life challenges successfully. All signs of good health. Vagal tone

can be improved through Yoga practices, such as lengthening exhalations, slow and mindful movements, restorative postures, meditation, and chanting.

Vagal tone is measured by determining heart rate variability with an *electrocardiogram*, which tracks variations in the heart rate during breathing. The heart rate of a healthy person shows good variability; it speeds up during inhalations and slows down during exhalations. Low heart rate variability, which may result from relentless overactivation of the sympathetic nervous system, has been related to systemic inflammation and increased risk of chronic illness, such as diabetes and heart disease, as well as psychological conditions including anxiety and depression. ❖

THE PSOAS, HEALTHY ORGANS, AND LYMPHATIC FUNCTION

In ancient Greece, the psoas was called "the origin or the womb of the kidneys," which was farsighted given what we now know about the fascial connections between them.[22] Some of the abdominal and pelvic organs, including the kidneys, rest on and are supported by the "shelf" of the psoas. Research has determined that most of the weight of these organs is borne by the psoas muscles and only 12 percent of the weight is borne by suspensory ligaments.[23] This intimate relationship means that the organs can be affected, positively or negatively, by the tone of the psoas. Excessive tension in the supportive psoas has the potential to transfer this tone to overlying organs. Increased tonicity in the organs can affect their movement and function. Our students have related remarkable resolution of health issues involving the digestive, urinary, and reproductive systems after working with the psoas, and we hope these anecdotal results will stimulate interest in research that connects the dots between psoas function and optimal organ function. For now, we are confident to say that a relaxed and engaged psoas can provide support for organs and contribute to healthy function by providing a rhythmic massage during walking and other movements.

Lymph vessels and nodes are located along the pathway of the psoas muscles. Not only does the rhythmical contraction and release of the psoas massage organs and contribute to their healthy function, but also the mechanical pumping action of a healthy psoas during walking and other activity moves lymph, blood, and intercellular fluid. Unobstructed flow of lymph and other fluids throughout the body is an important component of a healthy immune system.

❊ Key Concepts

▸ Much of the weight of the abdominal and pelvic organs is borne by the muscular shelf of the psoas.

▸ A tight psoas can affect the optimal function of organs.

▸ Lymphatic fluid is moved mechanically by the pumping action of a healthy psoas during walking and other movements. ❊

ENERGETIC ANATOMY OF THE PSOAS

In the West, we reduce the concept of center to the physical location of the center of gravity, generally located just anterior to the second sacral vertebra, at the midpoint between the pubic symphysis and the navel. In Asian traditions, the concept of center constitutes much more than a physical position. Known variously as the *hara, lower dan tien,* or "mind palace," learning to locate and refine the position of this locus point constitutes a way of being in the world whereby the human body acts as a conduit between the forces of heaven and earth. In these traditions, the hara or belly is considered a veritable reservoir of life force energy. When we are home and truly centered in this place, our inner being is in harmony with nature and the laws of nature.

In his engaging book, *Hara, The Vital Center of Man,* Karlfried Graf Dürckheim defines hara as an all-inclusive general attitude that enables a man or woman to open him- or herself to the power and wholeness of the original life force and to testify to it by the fulfillment, meaningfulness, and the mastery displayed in his or her life.[24] In a moving passage, he describes the depth with which this vital center operates.

> Whenever a physical performance results from the right use of Hara that is, using one's middle, all the organs work as if in play, functioning as a whole, accurately, and without straining. And, even in the smallest partial action, the great whole is at work. But the whole includes more than the powers comprehended and guided by the I. If the basic center, which releases the strength of the whole is missing, the limbs then have to be consciously directed by the will. The effect is uncoordinated, without inner flow. There is fatigue and cramp soon follows. This is true of every action demanding physical strength, carrying, pushing, pulling, speaking, singing, writing, typing, dancing, climbing, cycling, etc. . . . Whenever work is done from Hara, that is, with a tranquil I and with the strength rising from the vital center, the effort is reduced to a minimum because the movement occurs organically and is not executed by the I.

We believe the psoas plays a vital role in accessing this powerful energetic center. Streaming along both sides of the spine and connecting the spine and pelvis to the legs, a balanced psoas is one of the key determinants in being able to establish a neutral position of the pelvis—that is, neither tipped forward causing a spilling of the abdominal contents, or tipped backward causing a flattening of the lower back. A pelvis calibrated in this neutral position has the capacity to relay impulses from the legs through to the upper body and to moderate impulses from the upper body all the way down to the feet. When we witness the performance of a fine dancer, an accomplished martial artist, a bold equestrian, or any finely tuned athlete, we are seeing the results of this mastery of the body's energetic center (Illustration 20). It is also present in the calm imperturbability

of a monk seated in deep meditation and in the grounded stance of a leader able to inspire. In all these expressions of the energetic core, the body's center has an invisible magnetic pull toward the support of the earth, and the rebound of that force creates a seemingly effortless upward movement of the body into space. Many of the exercises and inquiries you will explore in this book will help you to consciously find and move from the support of this energetic center.

❀ Key Concepts

▶ Centering the body energetically connects you to wholeness: the earth underneath you, the life around you, the sky above you.

▶ Centering your structure is the foundation for energetic balancing.

▶ When movement is coordinated from the energetic center, it is effortless yet powerful. ❀

SUMMARY

Although the anatomy of the psoas and the interconnections between it and other structures in the body are indeed complex, paradoxically this complexity also points to the psoas as a unifying structure. Therefore, any work that you do to release, balance, and strengthen the psoas has the capacity to have far-reaching consequences. More simply stated, sorting out your psoas can sort out a lot of other issues in the body, sometimes phenomenally quickly and efficiently.

The intimate connection of the psoas to the spine should make it the go-to zone for addressing spinal tension, compression, pain, and movement limitations. Situated as it is near the diaphragm and heart, and underlying the abdominal and pelvic organs, returning the psoas to its rightful state of pliant elasticity can support improved respiration and heart function as well as other organic

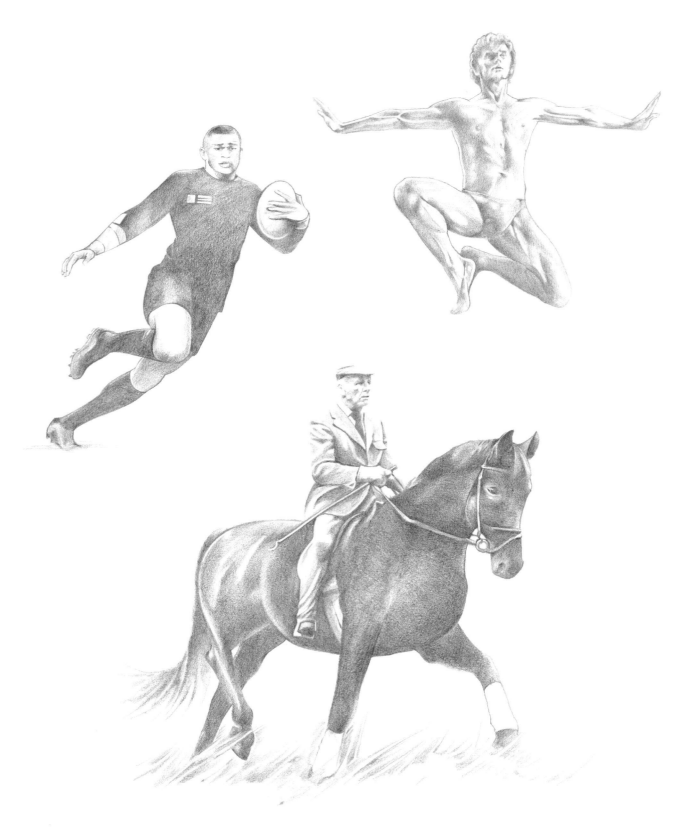

ILLUSTRATION 20: Supreme athletes attain mastery of the body's
energetic center through years of sustained practice.

processes, such as digestion and elimination. Its interconnections with the autonomic nervous system can help you target stress reduction and literally switch off debilitating chronic stress states. This allows your body to repair and restore itself.

Beyond these more objective physical outcomes, learning how to center your body can have a radical effect on your state of mind and emotions. With consistent practice, the psoas can become an accessible *touchstone* that can be used whenever you need to calm and steady yourself. Learning to register the sensations that precede the fight-or-flight response can help you to manage and transform emotions and habitual behavior patterns.

Your effort to more fully comprehend the anatomy of the psoas will give you deep insights into how the exercises in upcoming chapters can result in such noticeable changes. You will be able to integrate your intellectual understanding by more clearly imaging these structures and therefore develop the ability to deeply sense and directly feel the body from within.

Foundation Practices

INTEGRATING BREATH AND CORE ENGAGEMENT

IN MANY OF the inquiries and exercises in this book, you will find it beneficial to integrate your movement with your breath. In Chapter Two, you learned how the diaphragm and psoas share a mutual point of origin and how relaxation or tension can be transferred from one to the other. Learning to use your breath to relax and release is also the beginning of learning to use your breath to condense and engage your core muscles. Unfortunately for many people, the common command to "hold in the belly" crudely translates to "hold the breath." For other people, holding in the belly can be a completely unconscious ongoing activity. Certainly, if you try to engage your core through an isolated action of your outer abdominal wall, or through a static and unyielding abdominal contraction, you'll find it very difficult to breathe freely. In this chapter, you'll learn how to integrate breathing and movement so that you can consciously direct your breath depending on whether you want to relax and release, or whether you need to actively engage your core muscles for stabilization (while still breathing fully to support your activity). To achieve this, you'll need to distinguish between the two main kinds of breathing: Abdominal Breathing and Diaphragmatic Breathing. Once you have these skills under your belt, we will introduce you to Constructive Rest Position as well as variations that you can practice for specific structural issues. To prepare you for deeper work in the chapters to come, we will guide you step by step in locating, finding, and feeling the pathway of the psoas muscles.

ABDOMINAL BREATHING

The thoracic diaphragm (just above your waist) is designed to be the primary mover of the breath. This double-domed structure not only moves up and down but also can radically expand the rib cage to the sides of the body. As the diaphragm descends on an inhalation, it displaces the abdominal organs, causing a sequential wave through the abdomen that should go all the way down to the pelvic floor, resulting in a gentle downward swelling around the perineum (the area between the genitals and the anus). The abdominal wall will respond by *releasing outward* as the belly expands. During exhalation, the diaphragm ascends, and the abdominal organs naturally migrate upward. The upward ascent of the thoracic diaphragm draws the pelvic diaphragm upward, with the abdominal muscles *gently retracting toward the center* as the belly condenses. This natural mode of breathing is called Abdominal Breathing (also known as Belly Breathing) and is incredibly effective for releasing muscular tension and bringing awareness to the pelvic area. Use this type of breathing for the inquiries and exercises that help you soften, hydrate, release, and lengthen the psoas and spinal muscles. It also can help to release anxiety and emotional holding. But Abdominal Breathing is not the kind of breathing that supports your body in dynamic activity such as when you lift weight. Nor will Abdominal Breathing stabilize your body during sports such as skiing or horseback riding or enable you to move effortlessly from the ground to standing. Read on.

DIAPHRAGMATIC BREATHING

In Diaphragmatic Breathing, the expansion of the breath is directed consciously to the lower border of the rib cage. On an inhalation, the diaphragm descends and the rib cage broadens. Some health practitioners refer to Diaphragmatic Breathing as Horizontal Breathing, which aptly describes the directional orientation of this breath. During Abdominal Breathing, the abdominal wall relaxes completely, whereas in Diaphragmatic Breathing, the abdominal wall becomes actively engaged.[1] Looking down your torso, you will see the abdomen expand but to a much lesser degree

than in Abdominal Breathing. Your deliberate engagement of the abdominal wall acts like a corset, preventing the abdominal organs from spilling forward. The abdominal organs have to go somewhere: as they meet the resistance of a firm abdominal wall, the organs are displaced *to the sides* and *to the back* of the body. While Abdominal Breathing is like putting a sleeping bag in a large stretchy pillowcase, Diaphragmatic Breathing is like compacting that same sleeping bag into a small canvas duffel. This containment of the abdominal wall increases the pressure inside the abdomen (known as intra-abdominal pressure). The resulting increased compaction through the core of the body is one of the mechanisms that stabilizes the spine. This is why the diaphragm is considered to be a key player in the activation of the core muscles.

As a result of this slight resistance of the abdominal wall, the diaphragm has to work a little harder to descend during this type of breathing, which strengthens the diaphragm. Strengthening the diaphragm can improve breathing function allowing you to take deep, full, and complete inhalations and exhalations, which in turn maximizes oxygen uptake and carbon dioxide removal. Diaphragmatic Breathing turns the diaphragm into a star contributor to core stability.

While Abdominal Breathing creates a mental state that is relaxed and even a little sleepy, Diaphragmatic Breathing creates a clear, attentive, and ready-for-action state of mind. You will practice this kind of breathing when performing many of the strengthening inquiries and exercises in this book, and when you need a bit more oomph to support your activity or movement practice.

BREATH RESTRICTION

If your psoas muscles are tight, this may lead to a diminished movement of your thoracic diaphragm. This can lead to breathing that is either predominantly a movement of your lower abdomen or predominantly a movement of the secondary respiratory muscles high in the neck and chest. Some health practitioners refer to high chest breathing as Vertical Breathing, which aptly describes the "up and out" directional orientation of this way of breathing. When you place your hands around your lower ribs you will feel little or no movement of your ribs. That means the thoracic diaphragm is no longer working as efficiently as it could.

Shallow, low Abdominal Breathing tends to pair with a collapsed body posture and an overall depressed and lethargic demeanor. Upper chest or Vertical Breathing tends to pair with a hypertonic military posture, with excessive tension in the upper back, neck, throat, and jaw; and often accompanied by feelings of anxiety, tension, and hypervigilance. The following inquiries will help you find a middle ground.

⁝⁝ INQUIRY: *Activating Diaphragmatic Breathing*

In the following exercise, we are going to play a little trick on our body to "install" the precise movement of Diaphragmatic Breathing.[2] To begin, sit with crossed legs with the pelvis supported on a blanket or cushion (or sit on the edge of a chair with the feet wide apart) so your spine is erect. Begin by observing your breath just as it is. Bring your hands around your lower rib cage and notice whether it expands to the sides as you inhale or whether the rib cage has little or no movement. Now take a normal inhalation through your nose, then on your exhalation gently purse your lips and make a *WHO* sound (like the sound you hear when listening to a seashell). Imagine a candle flame just in front of you and that you are making your outgoing breath so gentle and smooth that it does not disturb the flame. Continue for ten breathes, breathing in through the nose and out through pursed lips. After ten breaths, let your breathing return to normal. Notice whether the quality of your breathing has changed. Has your exhalation become longer? Are your inhalations feeling fuller? Can you feel the thoracic diaphragm beginning to broaden the entire circumference of the rib cage?

Now complete another ten sets of the *WHO* breath. During this round as you exhale, notice that the action of making the *WHO* sound is subtly activating the abdominal muscles. This gentle activation of the abdominal muscles tends to increase the length of the exhalation. Taking a *full exhalation* tends to provoke a *full inhalation.* Notice that after switching on your abdominal muscles during the exhalation, they remained switched on during your inhalation as well. This subtle activation of the abdominal muscles during inhalation is a hallmark of the type of breathing that supports core stability. Abracadabra . . . you are now taking a Diaphragmatic Breath.

Make a habit of taking ten *WHO* breaths three times a day as a way to retrain yourself to breathe diaphragmatically and to generalize this breathing during all of your everyday activities. Practicing before each meal is a good way to install this precise movement. You can become even more focused in this practice by counting your breaths with the aid of your fingers: close your fingers into your palms and after each exhalation open one finger, starting with the little finger on your right hand and finishing with the little finger of your left hand. You'll be surprised how calm and steady your mind feels when you regularly complete this practice. ⁝⁝

Powerful Breath (*Ujjayi Pranayama*)

The pranayama technique of the Powerful Breath (*Ujjayi Pranayama*) often is engaged during active asana practice. This breath work will subtly switch on the abdominal muscles and support Diaphragmatic Breathing. Ujjayi involves a slight closure of the vocal cords, or glottis, at the base of the throat. When practiced sensitively, your breathing will sound like the echo of the ocean inside a seashell––a deep but soft "ssss" on the inhalation and an "hmm" on the exhalation. This type of breathing never should be forced so that you sound like Darth Vader: practicing in this exaggerated manner will only cause excessive tension.[3]

PRACTICES

Constructive Rest Position

Many of the inquiries and exercises in this book begin in Constructive Rest Position (CRP). As you will see, CRP can be an exceptional stand-alone practice for releasing the psoas and spine. You can use it for 5–15 minutes (or more) with amazing results. At first you may feel that "nothing is happening." We tell our students that when you put a cake in the oven you don't pull your cake out of the oven after 3 minutes and declare that something is wrong with the recipe because the batter is still wet. Just as it takes time for a cake to bake, it can take time for the body to unwind and release. When you come out of many of these positions, you may be surprised to discover just how much the body has changed during your seemingly uneventful stay. If you tend to be fidgety and impatient, set a timer and put on some quiet soothing music. Cover your eyes and ensure that you feel warm. A wheat bag warmed in the microwave for a few minutes and then laid over the abdomen, can work wonders to facilitate relaxation. Take a little time to become familiar with the particular variations of CRP that work best for your body. This is not only a *go-to* practice; it is a *go-back-to* practice if you are feeling discomfort of any kind. Enjoy.

❖ *Body Stories: Embodying Emotions*

While practicing a psoas release that involved her partner touching her upper thigh, Loralie felt her back muscles tighten with painful sensations radiating up her spine. She relayed this to the assistant teacher, who suggested she immediately return to Constructive Rest Position. Within a few minutes, the painful sensations abated accompanied by a spontaneous welling of emotion and a realization that the safe, yet intimate, touch of her partner had triggered memories of past sexual abuse. Surprisingly, as she rested in CRP, both the physical and emotional discomfort vanished within minutes. When Loralie decided she was ready to again try the assisted psoas release, she was delighted to feel a deep release along the entire length of her spine. ❖

Benefits

- Puts the body in an optimal position to release the psoas and spine.
- Alleviates compression in the lumbar spine and can release pressure in the sacroiliac joint.
- Calms the body, mind, and emotions while also promoting a sense of relaxed alertness.

Contraindications

- May be problematic for those with compromised disk integrity in the lower back.
- May be uncomfortable for those with inflammation in the sacroiliac joints or the lower back—try Variation A using the Muscle Release Ball (MR Ball).[4]
- If you have spondylolysis or spondylolisthesis, first try Variation D.

You'll Need

- A yoga mat covered with a wool or cotton blanket.
- A towel, washcloth, yoga belt, MR Ball, and a bolster depending on the variation you practice.

Why: CRP not only is the go-to position for releasing the psoas but also is an excellent foundation practice for rebalancing and lengthening the entire spinal column. It is one of the most powerful practices that we use for anyone with spinal discomfort. The careful placement of the legs establishes the skeleton as the primary support so that the deep core muscles can relax and release. The hip bones "plug into" the hip socket, and with the assistance of gravity, allow the whole length of the psoas to release the spine. The subtle relaxed alertness required to maintain the position of CRP represents a balance between relaxation and positive tension. This balances the three pillars of the nervous system—sympathetic (action and alertness), parasympathetic (rest and restore), and enteric (the brain in the belly).

How: To lie in CRP, place your feet far enough away from your buttocks that the upper and lower leg bones "rest against each other like cards" (Figure 1). In this position the rectus femoris (quadriceps) and the rectus abdominis (outer abdominal muscles) will be optimally relaxed. These two muscles are most likely to duplicate the action of the psoas. If your feet are too close to the buttocks, you will find that your upper thighs are unnecessarily tense and that the weight of your body primarily will be on the ball of your foot. If your feet are too far away from your buttocks, the abdominal muscles will be too engaged and the weight of the body primarily will be in the heel of the foot.

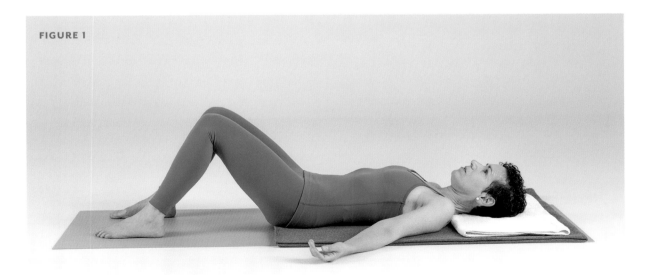

FIGURE 1

When the weight is balanced equally between the ball and heel of the foot, and you have some air space behind the knee, you are approaching the zone of an optimal CRP. Also check that the feet are hip-width apart; if the feet are too wide apart, the knees will fall inward; if the feet are too narrow, the knees will fall outward. Briefly, look down your torso and check that the thighs are in a parallel position and that the weight on your feet is balanced between the inside and the outside of the foot. Last, if you feel discomfort in your neck and it appears that your chin is higher than your forehead, place a folded towel under your neck and head until the forehead is *slightly* higher than the chin. Use as much towel support as is necessary to feel comfortable but do not use so much support that it causes the head to be raised significantly higher than the neck. Now relax for 5–15 minutes. When you are ready to come out of CRP, roll over to your right side and curl up to sitting.

Variations of Constructive Rest Position

Variation A—Psoas Awareness
with Muscle Release Ball: Resting in CRP, place a folded blanket or a half-deflated MR Ball under the pelvis so that the sacrum is fully supported. Place a folded yoga belt or thin washcloth at the

12th thoracic vertebra (T12), situated at the base of the rib cage just above your waistline (Figure 2). Ensure that the belt or washcloth is not too thick or it will be uncomfortable. Recall the origin of the psoas at T12 and the insertion at the lesser trochanters of the femurs. Imagine the 40-centimeter (16-inch) length of the psoas as a hammock that is suspended at one end by the lesser trochanters of the femurs while the base of the thoracic spine (T12) rests on the floor. Rest the hands on the upper abdomen. On each exhalation, imagine the hammock sagging a little closer to the ground. Visualize the diagonal pathway of the psoas from the front to the back of the body. Stay for 5–15 minutes. Carefully remove the MR Ball and washcloth and extend your legs along the floor. Notice whether you feel more space in the lower back and spine as a result of practicing this variation.

Variation B—Hyperlordosis
(Increased Lumbar Curvature): For some people with tight psoas muscles combined with an increased lumbar curve (hyperlordosis), it can feel more comfortable to raise the pelvis on a folded blanket (Figure 3). Alternatively, you can place a bolster against a wall and rest the balls of your feet on the bolster with the heels on the floor and the feet flexed at a 45-degree angle (Figure 4).

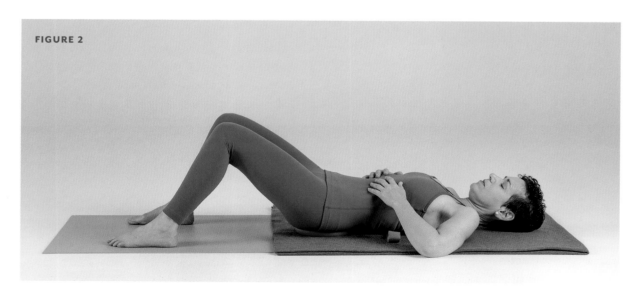

FIGURE 2

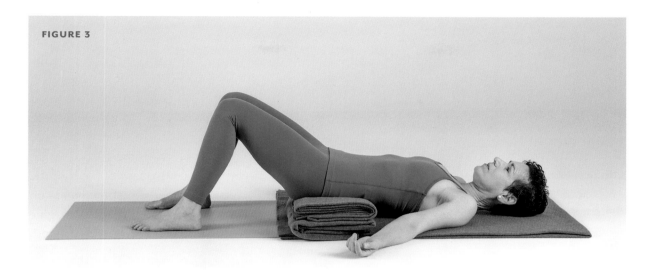

FIGURE 3

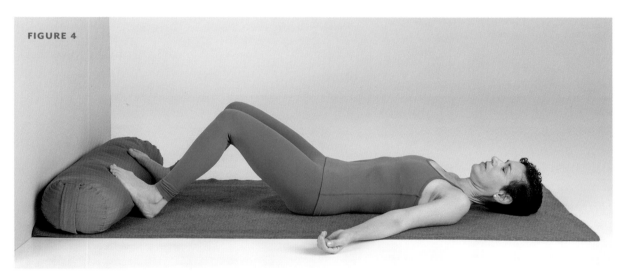

FIGURE 4

The supported flexion of the feet helps to shift the femur deeper into the hip socket, making it easier to release the psoas back toward the spine. You are not trying to flatten your lumbar curve or to press the back flat to the ground. Your aim is only to reduce the curvature (if it is accentuated) and restore the lumbar spine to a neutral position.

Variation C—Pelvic, Sacroiliac, and Lower Back Instability: Some individuals find that attempting to keep the thighs parallel creates profound tension. Tight psoas muscles and weak adductors (the muscles that assist inward rotation of the thighs) both can contrib-

ute to this tendency for the knees to splay apart. Using a cross-belt can secure the legs into a parallel position while at the same time stabilizing the pelvis and sacroiliac joints. The use of the cross-belt also can equalize the force between the left and right side of the pelvis.

To secure the cross-belt: Start with a 2½-meter (8-foot) yoga belt made of wide cotton webbing and a fastener at one end. Hold the fastener in your right hand in front of your right hip (Figure 5A). Now take the belt around the back of your upper thighs (just beneath the buttocks) (Figure 5B). Bring the belt across the left hip, crossing the

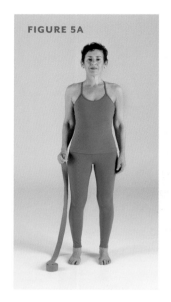

FIGURE 5A

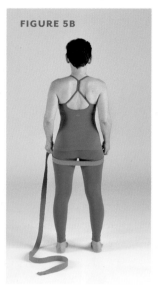

FIGURE 5B

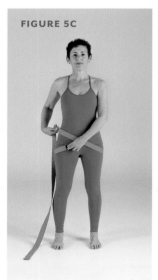

FIGURE 5C

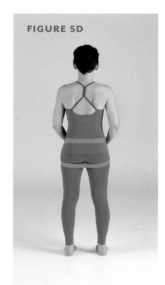

FIGURE 5D

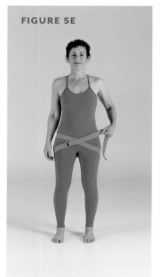

FIGURE 5E

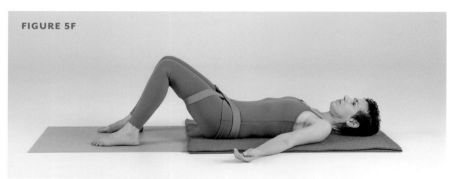

FIGURE 5F

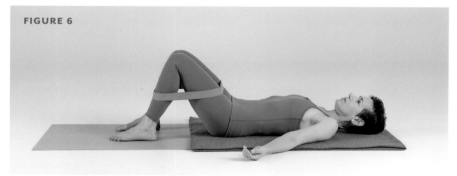

FIGURE 6

navel to the top of the right side of the pelvis (Figure 5C). Now take the belt around the back of the pelvis along the top rim of the pelvis, or slightly beneath the rim of the pelvis (Figure 5D). Do not put the belt across the back of the lumbar spine or waist. Finally, wrap the belt back to the front of the right hip and secure the tongue of the belt into the clasp. Pull until the belt feels snug (Figure 5E). As you lie in CRP, move the belt a little lower down on the thighs and tighten the belt until you feel that your legs are held in a parallel position (Figure 5F). Any outward pressure of the thighs against the belt only causes the cross-belt to draw the two sides of the pelvis more firmly together. Some people also find securing the belt around the shin and thighs works well to keep the thighs parallel and to give a sense of grounding through the legs and feet (Figure 6). You can use the cross-belt or shin-thigh belting technique during core stabilization exercises, in Bridge Pose (*Setu Bandhasana*; see page 125), or at any time when you want extra support for the pelvis, sacroiliac joints, or lower back. The cross-belt can also be effective during the practice of restorative postures such as Supported Bridge Pose (*Salamba Setu Bandhasana*) and for the practice of The Great Rejuvenator (*Viparita Karani*), in which the pelvis rests on a bolster with the legs up the wall, or the lower legs are supported on a chair (page 129).

Variation D—Spondylolysis or Spondylolisthesis: This position may be helpful for students with spondylolysis (degeneration of the vertebral structure) and spondylolisthesis (a forward slippage of the lower lumbar vertebrae). Some people with these conditions feel more comfortable when they raise their lumbar spine and trunk higher than their buttocks on a stack of blankets (Figure 7). This position elevates the upper lumbar and lower thoracic vertebrae and reduces shearing stress on the displaced lower lumbar vertebrae and disks. Raising the lumbar spine and trunk may seem counterintuitive, but we have had amazing success creating comfort in students with these conditions who previously have been unable to lie comfortably on the floor.

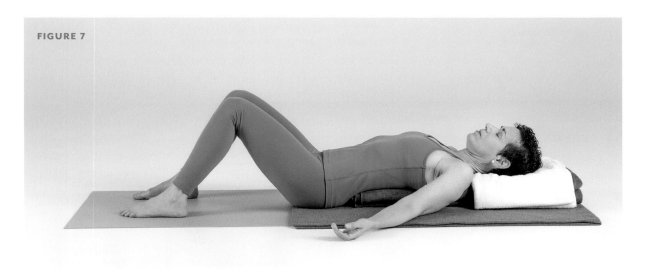

FIGURE 7

INQUIRIES: *Finding Your Psoas*

It is helpful to locate the psoas through touch. Developing a *felt sense* of the pathway of the psoas can help you to get a clear kinesthetic awareness of how to soften, lengthen, or engage this muscle and thus increase the benefits of many of the practices that follow. If you can feel it, you can heal it! Tracing the attachments and pathway of the psoas muscle can highlight your awareness of this deep abdominal muscle, but invasive palpation of the psoas is counterproductive and serves no useful purpose. Furthermore, manual deep palpation of the psoas can bruise muscle fibers and even damage arteries and internal organs. For these reasons, we suggest you decline any offers to have anyone massage your psoas unless trained and experienced in subtle release techniques.

If you've ever had a body worker massage a tight muscle too deeply, too quickly, or too specifically (poking with fingers or elbows), you'll know from experience that it results in defensive flinching and guarding. This is especially true of the psoas muscle because it is one of the first muscles in the body to contract during a fight-or-flight response. For this reason, approach tracing the pathway of your psoas with gentleness, sensitivity, and respect. You are *not* trying to put your fingers directly on the psoas muscle. It is buried under layers of tissue and organs. You simply are highlighting the presence of the psoas muscles in your mental landscape and then feeling the inferred movement when it is activated.

Give yourself at least 10–15 minutes for each side to create an unhurried and relaxed atmosphere while you learn to trace the pathway of these deep muscles. Always use the soft pads of the fingers to touch, never the fingertips, which can be too invasive. The psoas can be located easily when it is activated either with the breath or during the movement of hip flexion, or using both simultaneously.

Lie in CRP. If at any time during this exploration, you become agitated or you feel discomfort, stop immediately and return to the practice of Abdominal Breathing. It can be helpful to have an empty stomach, bladder, and bowel for this exploration. ⠿

⠿ Locating the Attachments

We'll start by simply identifying the location of the psoas attachments. It is important to do this inquiry one side at a time to increase the specificity of the experience in the brain. Begin with the right psoas muscle. To access the upper spinal attachments, place your left hand at the solar plexus, with the finger pads at your midline where the ribs join. Then move the fingers down and slightly to the right so they rest on the upper abdomen just below the ribs and approximately 4 centimeters (1-1/2 inches) from the midline. Under your hand, visualize the spinal attachments of the psoas on the transverse processes, bodies, and disks of the upper lumbar vertebrae. Imagine these upper fibers of the psoas filling with breath on your inhalations, and then softening and falling back into gravity to nestle along either side of the spine on your exhalations. Continue for several breaths.

The lower femoral attachments of the psoas are so deeply buried under layers of muscle that you can get only a rough idea of their location. In this inquiry, we will identify the landmarks that can help you to locate the psoas insertion. Place the finger pads of the right hand just below the groin crease so that the fingers touch the inner thigh area. Move the knee slightly to the side and gently feel the large tendon that pops up at the inner thigh. With a soft touch, explore the topography of this tendon by feeling its shape and density. This is *not* the psoas! It is only a landmark—the tendon of one of the large adductor muscles. Now realign your legs and move your fingers 8–10 centimeters (3–4 inches) laterally to palpate the large tendon situated in the middle of upper thigh just below the groin crease. Feel this tendon contract as you lift the right foot off the floor slightly. This also is *not* the psoas! Again, it is another landmark—the tendon of the rectus femoris of the quadriceps group. Remember that this is one of the more superficial muscles that can duplicate the action of the psoas. Slide your finger pads off the rectus femoris tendon into the valley between these two tendons and approximately 3–4 centimeters (1½ inches) below the groin crease. You are now touching the surface directly above the shared

FIGURE 8

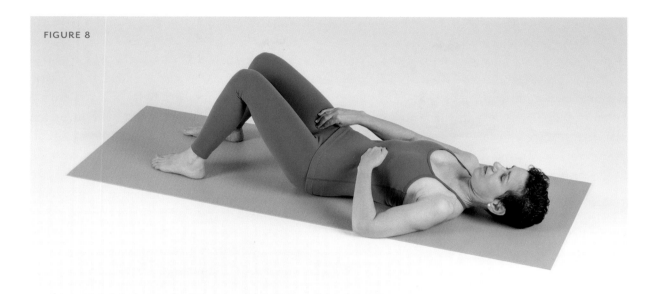

deep attachment for both the psoas major and the iliacus on the lesser trochanter of the femur (Figure 8). For our purposes, it is enough to be able to touch and visualize the approximate location of this attachment. Spend several breaths directing your breath into this area, imagining the psoas muscle filling with breath on your inhalations and softening on your exhalations.

Repeat the same practice on the left side. Then rest for a few moments and notice whether your perception of the location of the psoas muscles has been clarified.

Breathing Into the Psoas Muscles

Once again, let's start with the right psoas muscle. Gently place the palms of both hands on the right side of the abdomen so they rest on the pathway of the psoas. Visualize the weight of the 40-centimeter (16-inch) length of the right psoas slung like a heavy hammock between the upper and lower attachments. Using an Abdominal Breath, on an inhalation, imagine that the psoas is filling and expanding with breath like a balloon as it inflates. On your exhalation, imagine the psoas deflating, softening, and sinking a little deeper toward the earth and nestling alongside the spine. Extend the exhalation so it is longer than the inhalation. Continue this practice for several breaths until you can sense that the psoas muscle is calm and receptive.

Some people find it helpful to silently talk to the psoas in a reassuring way using phrases like "It's okay," "I'm here," or "You are safe now." It may be helpful to add the tactile cue of your hand gently stroking the length of the psoas in a soothing way. As you exhale, lightly stroke down the length of the psoas several times either with the fingers or with the full palm. Experiment to discover which type of touch feels calming and reassuring. Continue this practice for several breaths.

Repeat the same practice on the left side; then rest silently for several moments and notice whether you have a stronger felt sense of both the location and presence of your psoas muscles.

Accessing the Psoas with Diaphragmatic Breathing

Because the psoas and the diaphragm co-contract, the presence of the psoas is easily felt while practicing a Diaphragmatic Breath. When inhalation is deliberately initiated from the thoracic diaphragm, the emphasis of the movement is on the lateral broadening of the rib cage. You may want to place your hands on your lower ribs as you inhale and gently expand sideways into the firm pressure of your hands. Or you might imagine you have an elastic band wrapped around your lower rib cage, and with each inhalation, you expand into the circumference of the band. If tactile cues are helpful to you, wrap a yoga belt loosely around your lower rib cage. As you inhale, expand the breath to make contact with the belt.

Lie in CRP. Now recall the location of the right psoas muscle and its diagonal pathway from the solar plexus to the groin. Place your left hand on the upper attachment of the right psoas (as you did in the previous exercise).

Take a diaphragmatic inhalation, consciously expanding the ribs sideways and minimizing the movement of the breath in the abdomen and chest. The abdomen, which is soft, will expand with the breath, while the psoas, which is hard, will rise up from below to meet the finger pads. If you are unsure whether you are on the line of the psoas muscle, walk the fingers slightly medially or laterally to differentiate the softness of the abdomen and the hardness and vertical orientation of the psoas. You can gently move the finger pads from side to side to feel the underlying ropey texture of the psoas. Make sure that your touch is superficial. Take two more diaphragmatic breaths and feel the psoas contract and rise up on the inhalation then recede on the exhalation. ⁞⁞

Tracing the Psoas with Hip Flexion

For this inquiry, step your feet closer to your buttocks in CRP. If you are unsure whether you are feeling the contraction of the psoas muscle, while inhaling diaphragmatically (or suspending the breath after inhalation) lift the right foot off the floor approximately 5 centimeters (2 inches). The psoas will further contract and become more palpable as the hip bone flexes. Lower the foot back to the floor as you exhale. Repeat a few times until you think you may be feeling the psoas contract under your fingers. Remember to use a light touch.

Walk the finger pads approximately 3 centimeters (1 inch) down the length of the psoas muscle. Gently palpate the contraction of the underlying psoas muscle at that level for two or three diaphragmatic breaths. If necessary, confirm your location by lifting the foot off the floor to contract the psoas even more. If you experience any discomfort, lighten your touch. You want the psoas muscle to rise up to your fingers rather than pressing the fingers into the abdomen. Repeat this process of superficial palpation at several different levels along the course of the psoas. Walk your fingers down the stiff length of the muscle little by little taking three or four diaphragmatic breaths at each step. Continue until you reach the groin crease.

If you are unsure whether you are actually feeling the psoas, do not press more deeply into the abdomen. Rather, be more specific and precise with the diaphragmatic breath or with the location of your finger pads. If you suspect that you are feeling the psoas contract, you probably are. ⁞⁞

Body Stories: Learning To Be Gentle

Leah, a workshop participant, reported that accessing her psoas dramatically changed her life: "All my life I've been very hard on myself. When I feel my psoas muscles now, I feel a warmth and softening deep inside that reminds me to treat myself more gently."

Restoration

Even gently tracing the psoas can agitate a chronically contracted psoas muscle, so it is important to soothe it by returning to the breathing and stroking practices just noted. Spend at least 5 minutes calming your psoas muscles. If it is comfortable, turn over onto your belly and rest your forehead on crossed forearms. Stay in this position doing Abdominal Breathing for several breaths. Notice any feelings or sensations in the area of the psoas muscles. Alternatively, you may find it soothing to lie with your lower legs supported by a bolster.

No Pain Is Your Gain

With these basic foundation practices under your belt, you are now ready to explore the other inquiries and exercises in this book. Each time you enter a practice, notice whether it is best supported through Abdominal Breathing or Diaphragmatic Breathing. Feel whether particular movements are best practiced on an inhalation or exhalation. Also consider that the particular CRP that best suited you yesterday may not be the ideal fit today depending on what you are feeling in your body. Forget the cultural credo of "no pain, no gain." Pain is the body's way of saying, "Try another pathway." It is the clearest message the body can give you to alter your position and instead explore how "no pain can be your gain." Having an impeccably high standard for comfort will lead you toward the best alignment of your unique structure and move you ever closer to your true center.

CHAPTER 4

Soften and Hydrate

A HALLMARK OF ALL sound fitness routines is an initial period of gentle movements, usually referred to as the "warm-up." The goal of the warm-up is to lubricate the joints, pump fluid into the muscles, heat the body tissue, and awaken the senses in preparation for increasing range of motion. In any established dance studio, you will see even the most accomplished professionals beginning their routine with movements that involve swinging, rolling, pulsing, and oscillating, as well as more graduated versions of movements that will be expanded after the body has been thoroughly prepared. Similarly, in martial arts such as Tai Chi and Qi Gong, practitioners begin with movements that promote fluency and ready the body for more challenging practices. We refer to the warm-up in our protocol as a time to soften and hydrate the body tissue, which we view as qualitatively different than trying to stretch or strengthen.

THE IMPORTANCE OF WARMING UP

Unfortunately, many fitness regimens and many forms of Yoga do not incorporate this important phase of practice, but instead begin with static postures or sequences that immediately take the body into extreme ranges of motion. We tell our students that "just because you can, doesn't mean you should," and that seemingly innocuous movements like Upward Facing Dog (*Urdhva Mukha Svanasana*) represent an extreme backbend for the spine. Even a young and flexible professional dancer knows that starting her day with a *grand jeté* (a leap in the air with the legs in the splits) could be career ending. Whatever your practice may be, consider how a gentle and thorough warm-up period can enable your body to move with ease and provide some insurance that you will be able to continue to enjoy long into the future the activities, sports, and hobbies that give you pleasure.

This chapter will introduce you to several practices that can help you to soften and hydrate the psoas muscles. These practices can be

57

incorporated into almost any fitness or movement regimen. Consider that approaching your body with gentleness is truly advanced Yoga practice—increased range of motion should be a consequence of easeful and joyful movement, not a result of force and strain.

⁘ INQUIRIES: *Regular Walking* ···

One of the easiest ways to warm and soften your psoas muscles (and the rest of your body) is to make walking a part of your regular routine. By walking, we are not referring to the stiff and robotic power walking now so common on our thoroughfares, but rather walking with a relaxed and free-swinging rhythm through both the arms and legs. When the arms and legs swing freely, a natural counter-rotation occurs between the rib cage and the pelvis: this beautiful spiraling movement is the hallmark of contralateral movement. In the contralateral movement of walking, the reach of the arm draws the opposite leg forward. The left arm connects *through the core* to the right leg; the right arm connects *through the core* to left leg. If you pause for a moment midflight in your walk (left arm and right leg forward, right arm back) you will feel a rotation through the middle of your body. This contralateral movement of walking connects your oppositional limbs through a diagonal pathway that has its nexus in the core of the body.

Start by walking on flat ground. Visualize your legs beginning from the top of the psoas at the 12th thoracic vertebra (T12) and initiate each step by swinging the leg from this point. Sense the movement of the psoas as it alternates between shortening and condensing as you flex the hip bone and lift the foot, and lengthening as you place the foot on the ground. Feel the sequential flow of movement from the push off from the ball of the back foot up the leg into the pelvis and spine, creating a slight extension through the lower back. As the leg swings forward and the heel strikes, the pelvis and lumbar spine move into slight flexion. Notice the undulating nature of the movement: the wave of extension moving up the spine on push off, followed by the wave of spinal flexion as the psoas contracts to lift the foot and swing the leg forward.

You may wish to return to walking after practicing many of the exercises in this book. Stroll around the room for a few moments and notice whether you feel greater ease and fluency in your gait. ⁘

⁘ *Pulsing the Psoas* ··

When the psoas is functioning optimally, a clear impulse relays from the feet through the legs into the pelvis and onward to the spine. You can first test this relay while in Constructive Rest Position (CRP) by gently pressing your feet into the ground and observing whether the impulse goes through a neutral pelvis and spine all the way to the head. Then quicken your pace until you have an easy oscillatory movement that pulses back and forth from head to toe. In many people, this sequential flow of force is blocked through the intercession of two muscles: the rectus femoris (quadriceps) and the rectus abdominis (outer abdominal muscles). If you recall from the anatomy section (Chapter Two), we call these muscles "superficial duplicators" because they can accomplish some of the actions of the psoas but with far greater effort. If you have come to rely exclusively on these more superficial muscles, you will try to initiate the relay by tightly contracting your thighs or by gripping the abdominal wall and buttocks. What will occur in each instance is a mechanical up-and-down thrust of the pelvis (the "honeymoon thing" as we like to call it to bring a little humor into the equation). Initiating the movement from the abdominal muscles and buttocks is a clear sign that you tend to overuse your superficial duplicators. Having an assistant or helper bring their fingers around the back of the top of the calf muscles and gently pulse (while you receive the impulse passively), may help you learn how to relax these superficial muscles and instead feel the relay of the impulse into the psoas (Figure 9). Continue pulsing for 3–5 minutes, taking small pauses if necessary. Once you've completed the basic practice, extend your legs out and relax. Many people feel a tingling, shimmering sensation throughout the body, as if the cells literally are humming. All tissues in the body love this jiggling movement, especially the joints. You also may notice an appreciable difference in your energy levels. ⠆

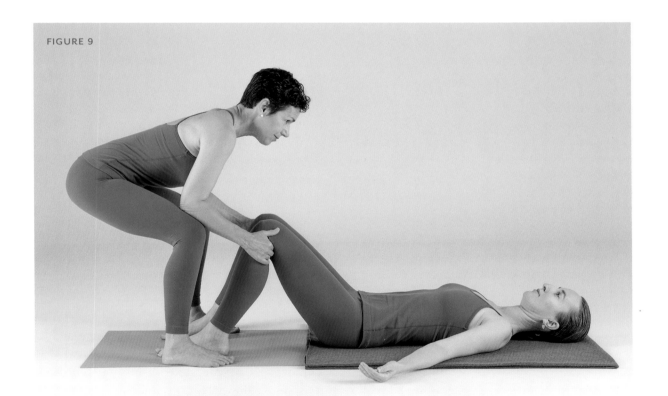

FIGURE 9

❖ Body Stories: The World of Walking

The next time you are in a busy public place, sit for while and watch the way people walk. Some people hold the upper body rigid or maintain a completely fixed spine, which inhibits the breath and the action of the arms and legs. Others swing their arms and legs as if their limbs were "taped" on at the shoulders and hips, with no connection to the core. Commonly, you may see "fitness" walkers, with their upper body charging ahead of the lower body. Or you may observe one side of the body pivots around the center so that walking becomes homolateral (left arm and left leg together), like a camel. Especially notice those whose walk is initiated from the knees with the trunk tipped forward. This is a strong indicator of a chronically contracted iliopsoas, and it often is seen in seniors as the precursor to hip replacement surgery. Can you identify any of these patterns in your own way of walking? ❖

PRACTICES

Hydrating the Psoas and Spinal Muscles

Benefits

- Hydrates the psoas and spinal muscles and increases differentiation of movement between individual segments of the spinal column.
- Improves lymphatic drainage as well as flow of fluid into and out of internal organs.
- Alleviates fatigue and promotes a sense of alertness.

Contraindications

- Oscillation while lying supine can be problematic for some but not all people with compromised disk integrity in the lower back.
- People with advanced osteoporosis or existing fractures of the spine should avoid doing this practice with the towel pressing on the vertebrae. You may be able to use very soft foam balls placed either side of the spine instead. If in doubt, consult with your health practitioner or a qualified Yoga therapist.

You'll Need

- A yoga mat and blanket: arrange these so that *only* your feet are on the mat and the rest of your body is on the blanket.
- A thin hand towel rolled into a cylinder no more than 3 centimeters (1 inch) in diameter. Secure the hand towel with three rubber bands, in the middle and at both ends.
- A folded towel under the neck and head so that the forehead is level with the chin.

Why: Most people store deeply held tension throughout the back. This tension is rarely alleviated through doing static Yoga postures. Sometimes muscles have become so densely compacted that attempting to lengthen them by stretching only serves to evoke a kind of rubber band pullback effect. The more you pull on the muscle fiber, the more it pulls back against your efforts. When you feel this kind of tension in your body, it's important to spend a little time softening and

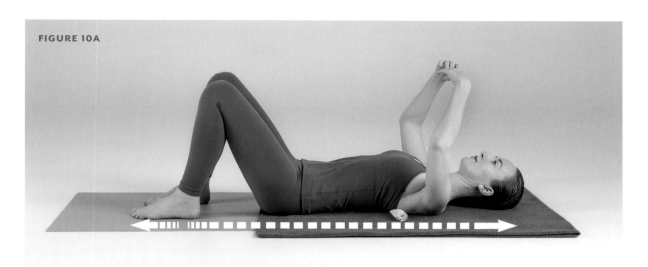

FIGURE 10A

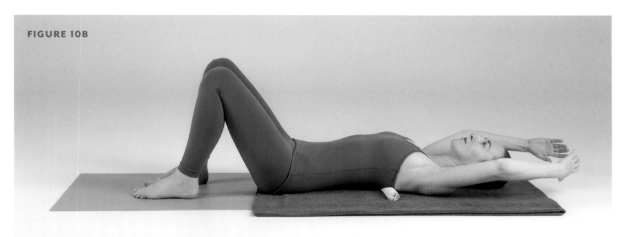

FIGURE 10B

hydrating the tissue before you attempt other practices. When your muscles lack fluidity, gentle pulsation can hydrate and lubricate the muscular tissue so that it is more amenable to lengthening.

How: Having tested your alignment in the previous practice, you now can continue with a more specific release for your entire spine. Start by lying in CRP once again. Place the rolled-up hand towel under your thoracic spine so that it is level with the top of your shoulder blades. Extend your arms above your chest with the elbows bent and the wrists and fingers dangling loose and relaxed (Figure 10A). Begin pulsing from your feet to your head. You will feel a specific oscillation around that particular vertebral segment. Now

add a movement of your arms. Starting with the arms over the chest, slowly extending the arms over the head without attempting to straighten or stretch them (Figure 10B). This movement will bring the spine into a very slight extension (back bending). Then slowly return the arms back to the starting position. This movement will bring the spine into slight flexion (forward bending). Then with the arms at chest height open the left arm to the side and turn your head to the left. The right elbow will bend with the hand touching the sternum (Figure 10C). This movement will rotate the spine. Continue to pulse from feet to head, taking several passes through the movement: arms overhead, back to center, and then turning left and right. While the whole spine is being moved sequentially into extension, flexion, and rotation, the individual segments of the spine that are positioned over the towel will receive a more specific release. Some people find it challenging to coordinate the pulsing while moving. If you get confused, just go back to pulsing while keeping the spine in a neutral position. If your arms or legs get tired during the practice, pause until you are ready to continue.

After several passes through the movement

sequence, pause and adjust your body so that the towel is now a little lower on the spine. Pulsing from feet to head, take several passes through the arm movements, and then when you are ready, adjust and move the towel a little lower again. When you eventually reach the lower back you'll find that the lumbar curvature (the hollow between the lower back and floor) makes it difficult to feel the towel against the spine. For this part of the spine, draw the knees gently into the

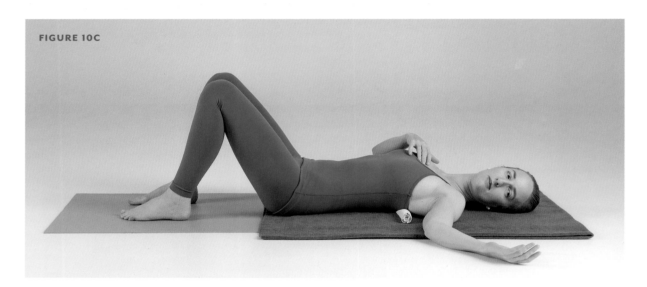

FIGURE 10C

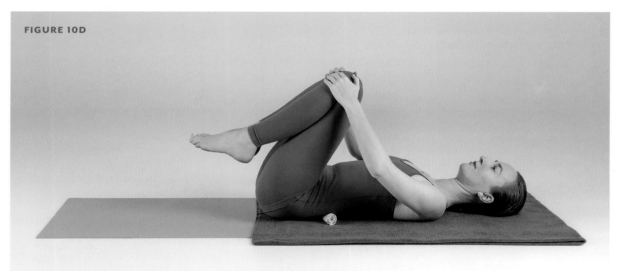

FIGURE 10D

chest, then while holding onto the knees, gently pulsate these lower segments by jiggling the knees forward and back (Figure 10D). Do not try to press your lower back into the floor. Try to keep the curvature of your lumbar spine neutral.

As you progress down the back, you may find that segments of your spine feel "glued together." Instead of having a differentiation of movement at each vertebral segment, it will feel like several vertebrae or even whole sections of the spine are moving as one block. The muscles in these areas of the back may feel more like bone than muscle. Spend a little more time pulsing on these seg-

ments, but don't become more aggressive with the pulsations as you may bruise the tissue. It is better to practice a little every three days than to forcefully press on that tight spot.

When you reach the top rim of the pelvis, place the feet back on the floor in CRP. The final position of the towel should be across the back of the pelvis and sacrum in line with the anterior superior iliac spine in the front (the prominent hip bones at the front of the pelvis) (Figure 10E). This is a powerful position for releasing compression in the sacroiliac joint.

Finally, every few pulses walk the feet away

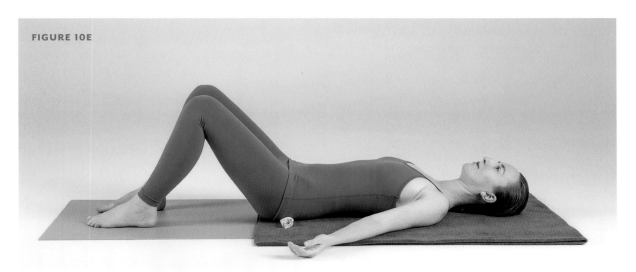

FIGURE 10E

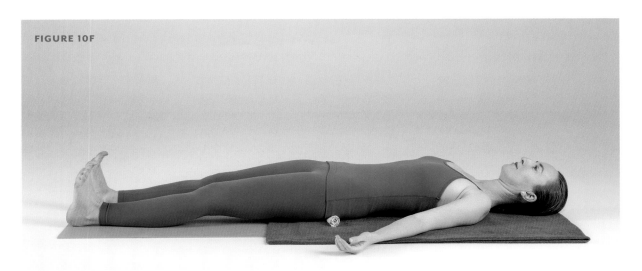

FIGURE 10F

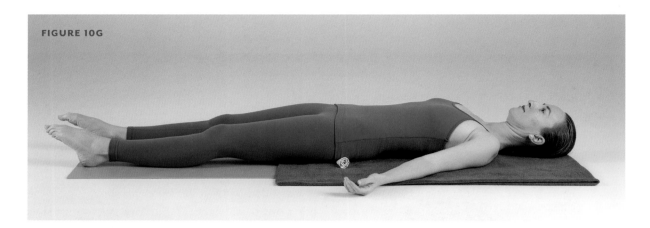

FIGURE 10G

from the buttocks. Eventually, the legs will be straight, and you will be pulsing by alternatively flexing and extending the heels (Figures 10F and 10G). Continue pulsing in this position for at least one minute. Then completely relax and notice how you feel physically and energetically as a result of this practice.

Prone Half-Butterfly with Muscle Release Ball

Benefits
- Softens and releases the deep insertion points of psoas major and iliacus muscles.
- Helps to restore the neutral position of the pelvis and lumbar spine.
- Alleviates compression in the lumbar spine and can release pressure in the sacroiliac joint.
- Reduces hyperlordosis.

Contraindications
- People with hypermobile sacroiliac joints should be careful not to overinflate the Muscle Release Ball (MR Ball)[1] and thus cause an excessive lift on one side of the pelvis.
- If this position does not feel comfortable in your groin, sacroiliac joint, or lower back, it is inappropriate for you to practice at this time.

You'll Need
- A yoga mat covered with a wool or cotton blanket.
- A bolster.

- An MR Ball, inflated to roughly one-third to one-half capacity.

Why: If your psoas muscle feels more like bone than muscle, and if you find lunge positions painful and result in little change, it's likely that your psoas is uninterested in releasing until it has had a chance to soften. Furthermore, once the psoas has gone into lock-down mode, postures that are intended to release your groin instead result in the lumbar spine hinging anteriorly and thus only accentuating the pull on the lower back. Opening the deep attachment points of the psoas at the hip can radically reduce this tendency to hinge in the lower back and bring the pelvis into a neutral position. Attaining a centered pelvic position is the most important component of attaining optimal and easeful posture.

How: Place a bolster along your blanketed yoga mat or carpet. Lie prone on the bolster with your lower abdomen and trunk supported by the bolster, with your legs resting on the floor. Flex the right leg 30–45 degrees at the hip resting the inner knee on the floor in a frog-like position. If necessary, decrease the angle of the thigh and knee so that you are comfortable throughout your inner groin and sacroiliac joints. Place an MR Ball, inflated to one-third to one-half capacity, so that the inside edge touches the midline of the pubic bone and the bulk of the ball is in the groin space (Figure 11A, close up). If the two sides of the pelvis feel radically uneven, further deflate the MR Ball. Drape your body over the ball and consciously give your body weight to the floor on progressive exhalations (Figure 11B). Taller people may find it more comfortable to have the sternum on the edge of the bolster and the forehead supported on the floor with a towel (Figure 11C). Stay for 5–7 minutes and then remove the MR Ball and release both legs. Lie for a moment on your belly. Notice whether you feel any difference between

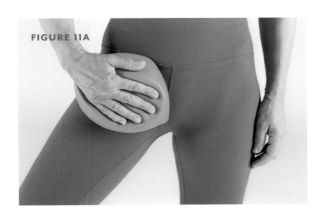

FIGURE 11A

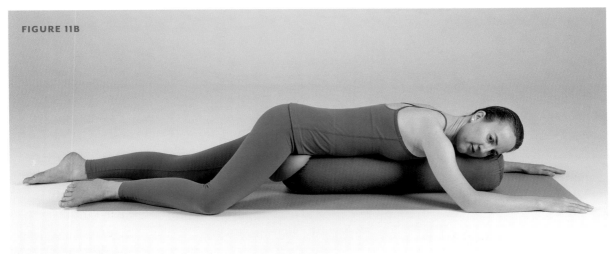

FIGURE 11B

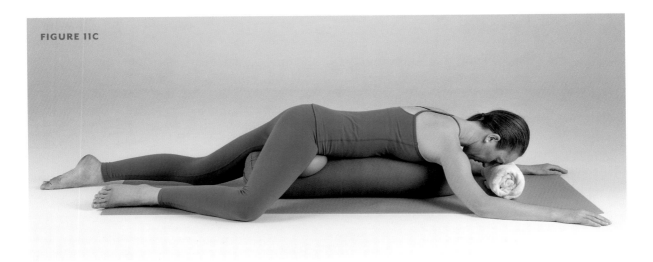

FIGURE 11C

the left and right groin. Then lie on your back and observe whether you feel one side of the back is now longer than the other. Now repeat the exercise on the left side.

Prone Half-Butterfly with Hip Slides

Benefits
- Softens and releases the insertion points of psoas major and iliacus muscles.
- Increases hip mobility.
- Helps to restore the neutral position of the pelvis.

Contraindications
- People with groin injuries should be cautious.
- People with hip dysplasia or hip replacement should consult with their health professional.
- If this position does not feel comfortable in your groin, sacroiliac joint, or lower back, it is inappropriate for you to practice at this time. Discomfort usually is the result of very limited movement within the hip socket itself; in these instances, it is better to first practice more gentle opening movements in a supine position (see Chapter Eight, pages 137–142, to learn a series of gentle hip mobilizing exercises).

You'll Need
- A yoga mat and blanket situated on a wood, tile, or linoleum floor (if you only have a carpeted practice area, place a sheet of paper or a plastic garbage bag under your knee so that it can slide easily on the carpet).
- A soft hand towel.
- An MR Ball, one-third to one-half inflated.

Why: This movement deepens and amplifies the effects of the previous exercise, creating even greater mobility.

How: Lie prone with the right leg flexed 45–90 degrees at the hip with the inner knee resting on a cushioned surface such as a folded soft towel. Place a deflated MR Ball under the groin as described in the previous exercise. If necessary, decrease the angle of the hip and knee so that you are comfortable throughout your groin and sacroiliac joints. Make sure your knee can easily slide along the floor, and if necessary, place a plastic bag or sheet of paper under the knee to facilitate glide

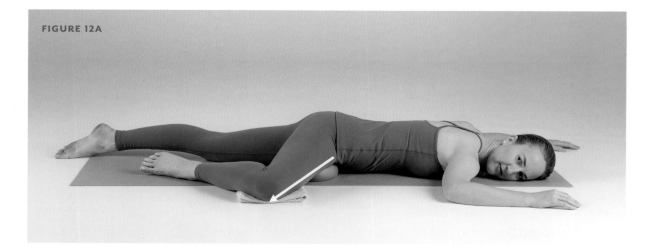

FIGURE 12A

of movement. Very gently slide the knee farther out to the side (the femur migrates out of the hip socket) so that the groin comes closer to the floor (Figure 12A). Then slide the knee back toward the groin (femur feeds back into the hip socket) to release the pressure on the groin (Figure 12B). In this position, a small hollow area should exist between the groin and floor. You can coordinate the movement with your breath by inhaling as the knee slides toward the midline and exhaling as the knee moves away from the midline. Continue for ten or more passes through the movement, being careful not to forcefully press the groin into the floor. Trust that the movement itself gradually will create the opening and release. After several minutes, remove the MR Ball and lie prone with both legs straight for a few moments. Then lie on your back and notice whether you detect any appreciable difference between your left and right sides. Now repeat the exercise on the left side.

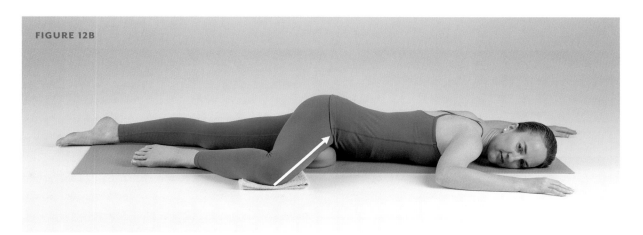

FIGURE 12B

Upward Puppy Spirals

Benefits

- Creates space between the spinal vertebrae.
- Hydrates through a "sponging" action of the psoas and spinal muscles.
- Prepares the body for deeper movements of extension.

Contraindications

- People with hyperlordosis should be cautious and practice the movement low to the floor.
- People with spondylolysis or spondylolisthesis should be cautious.

You'll Need

- A yoga mat and blanket to cushion your hips.

Why: Many Yoga methods such as *Ashtanga* Yoga and other styles of flowing postural sequences (known as *Vinyasana*), use the Sun Salutation (*Suryanamaskar*) as a core practice, often offered at the beginning of a session. We have found that many of our students compress and irritate their lower backs in the first few minutes of such classes through the extreme extension required to perform Upward Facing Dog Pose (*Urdhva Mukha Svanasana*). The rest of the practice is spent repairing the damage or in continuing discomfort. If the psoas and back muscles are tight, you will hinge in the most vulnerable segments of your spine—that is, between the 5th lumbar vertebra (L5) and the sacrum, and between the 1st lumbar vertebra (L1) and the rib cage—resulting in compression and discomfort in your back. In this variation, the emphasis is on lateral extension (side bending and rotation) and spiraling (which distributes movement over the entire spinal column and multiple planes of movement). Lateral extension allows you to open one side of the body at a time and also loosens the deep intervertebral muscles of the back. In this exercise, as one side of the psoas elongates, the other side shortens. The alternating movements of compression and decompression rehydrate the extensive psoas fascia. As these muscles loosen and warm, the spine naturally elongates, enabling deeper levels of extension. After warming the body through progressive cycles of this sequence, you may be surprised at how easily you can extend your spine without experiencing compression or discomfort. How differently the body responds when we prepare it well.

Practicing small degrees of extension against gravity is an excellent way to strengthen the muscles in the back that minimize kyphosis and that help to maintain lifelong erect posture.

How: Begin by lying prone on the floor resting on your forearms. Turn the forearms outward about 30 degrees (Figure 13A) Slowly turn your head to the right to look toward your right foot. As you

do so, your right thigh will turn outward. Then turn to look over your left shoulder to look back at the left foot. Gradually deepen the reach of your side bending so that your right knee bends as you look to the right side. You will be resting on the inside of the foot with the right foot in line with the right sitting bone (Figure 13B). To move to the other side, push off through the ball and toe of the right foot and gradually straighten the right leg until you are flexed to the left side, left knee bent. Feel that as you turn to the right you are anchoring the left groin and elongating the left psoas. As you turn to the left, anchor your right groin and elongate the right psoas. Move fluidly side to side for five to seven cycles.

On your next pass to the right side, extend your left arm on the diagonal along the floor over your head (Figure 13C). Roll onto the outside of your left shoulder and slowly bring the right arm across the sternum and out to the side, turning to look at your hand (Figure 13D). Reach out through the right arm as you counter-rotate back through the right knee. Do not jam your right knee to the floor, but rather allow it to come away from the floor as much as is necessary to bring your right shoulder onto the floor (Figure 13E, shown from other side for clarity). Then reach your right arm like the hand of a clock over your head, as you simultane-

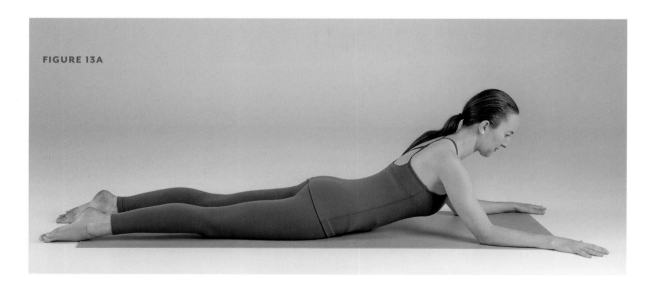

FIGURE 13A

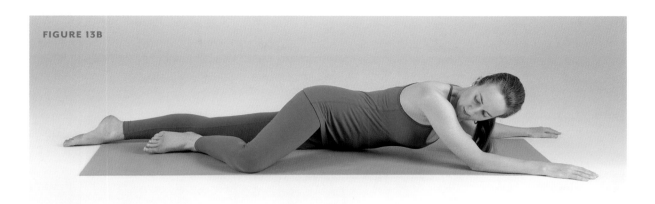

FIGURE 13B

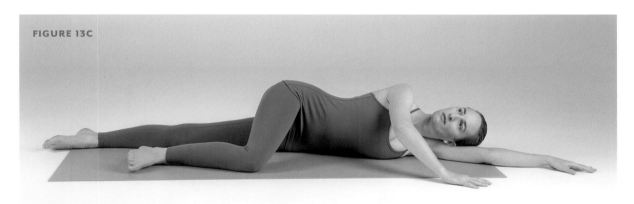

FIGURE 13C

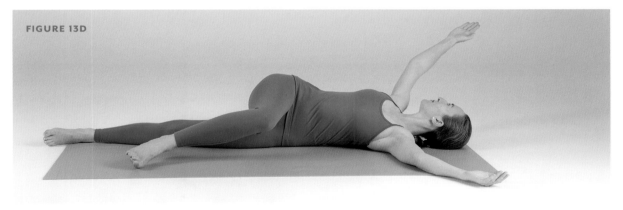

FIGURE 13D

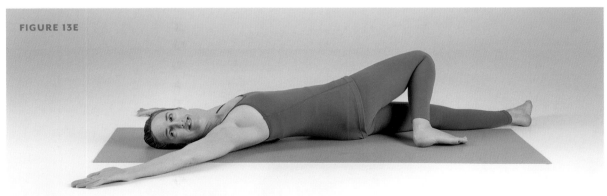

FIGURE 13E

ously reach through the right leg to spiral back onto your belly (Figure 13F, shown on left from behind). Return to the starting position (Figure 13A). Now repeat the sequence on the other side.

Practice for at least five cycles, alternating left and right sides. Notice that each time you return to the Upward Puppy Spiral position, your upper back, neck, and head have come a little farther away from the floor. As your back begins to accommodate this greater level of extension, explore slowly lifting the elbows off the floor and coming up into a modified Cobra Pose (*Bhujan-*

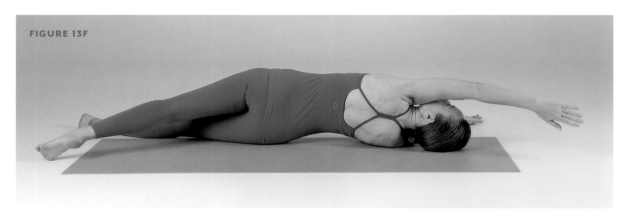

FIGURE 13F

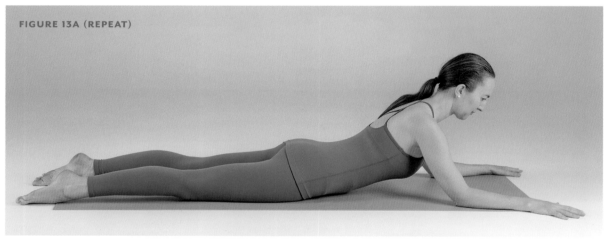

FIGURE 13A (REPEAT)

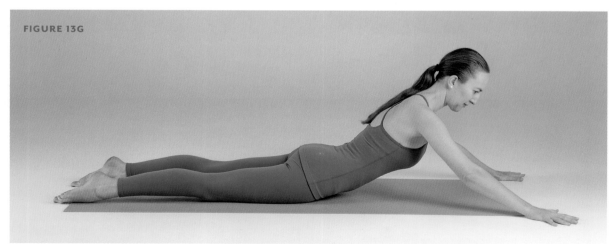

FIGURE 13G

gasana; Figure 13G). Make sure that your forearms are turned out at least 30 degrees.[2] If you feel any compression or discomfort in your back, slide your hands farther away from your body to mod-ulate the degree of extension (Figure 13H). A tiny extension accomplished without pain is better for your body than one hundred extreme backbends performed with strain.

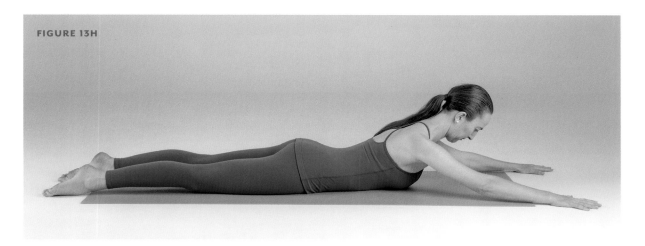

FIGURE 13H

Downward Facing Corpse Pose (*Adho Mukha Savasana*)

Benefits
- Releases the spinal muscles.
- Tones the internal organs.
- Calms and sedates the nervous system.

Contraindications
- None.

You'll Need
- A bolster.
- Two blankets.
- A bath towel.

Why: Lying prone for relaxation puts gentle pressure on the internal organs and stimulates their function while simultaneously releasing tension in the broad muscles along the back of the body. Many of our students find that this variation of Corpse Pose (*Savasana*) is a much more effective position for relaxation than lying supine. However, some people feel claustrophobic and uncomfortable lying prone. If you fall into the later category, simply roll onto your back and enjoy your relaxation supine.

How: Place a bolster lengthwise along a cushioned yoga mat. Fold a blanket to the width of the space from your pubic bone to your navel and place it across the bolster. Now lie on the bolster with your sternum on the edge and adjust the folded blanket so that it is under your abdomen. The sacrum should be slightly higher than the tail—adjust the folded blanket until you find a comfortable position. Let your knees turn slightly outward and move your elbows level with your shoulders, forearms at right angles. Place a folded towel under your forehead. Your head and neck should be aligned with the rest of your spine (Figure 14A).

If you have a hyperlordotic back, you may need to use several folded blankets placed along the length of the bolster to raise your torso. This added height will reduce the lumbar curvature (Figure 14B).

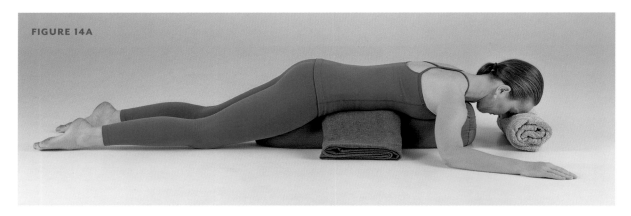

FIGURE 14A

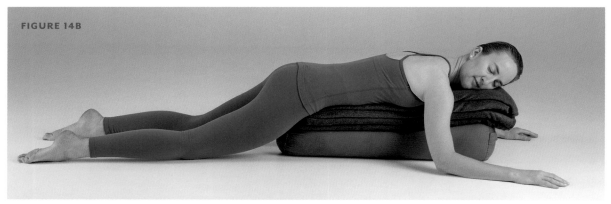

FIGURE 14B

PRACTICE SUMMARY

- Regular Walking
- Hydrating the Psoas and Spinal Muscles
- Prone Half-Butterfly with Muscle Release Ball
- Prone Half-Butterfly with Hip Slides
- Upward Puppy Spirals and Modified Cobra Pose
- Downward Facing Corpse Pose

The exercises offered in this chapter can become lifelong friends. After a long period of sitting or driving, a 10-minute session of Hydrating the Psoas and Spinal Muscles is an exceptional way to release tension in the back. Students who once had chronic back pain use this practice two to three times a week to maintain spinal comfort. The Prone Half-Butterfly has become a first line of defense for those with sacroiliac, sciatica, and lower back issues. And many of our students who previously endured pain and compression in

every single Sun Salutation no longer have these issues as long as they begin by thoroughly preparing with the Upward Puppy Spiral.

All these movements and supported restorative positions help to warm, soften, and increase tissue fluidity in the psoas so that movement (and stress) can be distributed over a greater portion of the whole spine. You also may notice that this fundamentally gentle approach helps you to soften in other ways. Letting go of striving and the effort to "get somewhere" enables the mind to relax in the moment. By relinquishing self-coercion, tender emotions that have been buried can now safely arise. Becoming centered is no longer something you need look for, but rather is something that is innately available to you the moment you turn inward.

CHAPTER 5

Release and Lengthen

HOW DID IT GET SO TIGHT?

W HAT CAUSES the psoas to become so tight in the first place? We don't have one simple answer to this question as causes can vary from individual to individual. What we do know, however, is that people are sitting for increasingly long periods of time, and this not only is detrimental to structural integrity but also can have serious health consequences.[1] Not only are we a society of sitters, whether in the car, at the office, or at home on the couch, we do not sit well. In fact, we rarely sit in a "self-supported" fashion, that is, without leaning against something, whether that something is the back of a chair, car seat, or a wall. Furthermore, we rarely vary our sitting position from the common chair sit (often done with crossed legs), which puts the hips and the psoas into a chronic position of flexion. Any position that is repeated over and over again has the potential to cause structural imbalances, and none more so than poor sitting habits.

Sitting crossed-legged on the floor with the pelvis slightly elevated so that the knees are lower than the hips (as demonstrated by anyone adept at meditation) has a different effect on the psoas, as does kneeling on a cushion with the back erect. And although we don't recommend sitting in any position for long stretches of time, self-supported sitting such as on a large exercise ball, on the edge of a chair or bench, or crossed-legged on the floor with support under the pelvis, stimulates the core muscles to engage. In fact, the more often you sit, stand, and move in a self-supported fashion, without leaning or collapsing into an external support, the faster you will build long and strong core muscles. What we practice, we get good at—the more you move with good posture, the easier it becomes for this to be the norm.

Notice that most of the psoas releases in this book involve extension of the groin or lumbar spine. This is the most obvious counter movement to balance long periods of flexion. Even simply standing and walking about for several minutes every hour can alleviate a chronically tight psoas, as can bringing your leg up onto the seat of your chair and taking a standing lunge.

If through necessity, you have a job that involves sitting, consider getting up frequently to walk and move about. Many companies are now offering standing desks in response to increasing concerns about the health consequences of long periods of sitting. If you have the privacy to lie down for 10–15 minutes, consider using Constructive Rest Position (CRP) as an alternative to your coffee break so that the spine and psoas can release.

Because everyday activities tend to create tightness in the psoas, learning how to release the deep psoas muscles can reap profound rewards, leading to graceful posture, greater ease in the spine, and better balance and coordination. Releasing the psoas also lays the foundation for building functional core strength that can support your daily activities so that you can sit without discomfort, walk fluidly, and lift weight, such as your groceries or a heavy wheel barrow, without putting stress on your spine.

At the same time, the anatomy of the psoas makes releasing this deep muscle a little tricky. With the origin of psoas major arising at the juncture between the base of the rib cage and the lumbar spine, a tight psoas can cause you to hinge

through this vulnerable segment of the back. For this reason, in some of the exercises that follow, you will need to consciously stabilize the insertion point of the psoas so that this part of the spine remains still and acts as an anchor point, enabling the rest of the psoas to elongate. In other exercises, you may need to create a dynamic tension and elongation between the two ends of the muscle— for example, anchoring the groin in Cobra Pose (*Bhujangasana*) as you slowly move the spine into extension. If at any time you feel compression, discomfort, or sensations that you have come to know as warning signals from your back, immediately modify your position. This could involve reducing the degree of spinal extension (e.g., not coming up as high in a movement such as Cobra) or lowering the height of your support (e.g., using a smaller bolster). If you have an instructor, ask for assistance. If you are still uncomfortable, come out of the position and return to CRP or any position that alleviates your discomfort. Some of the practices in this chapter may not be suitable for you at this time, but keep in mind that as your body opens, you may be able to do them safely in the future.

We recommend practicing one or two releases within your routine rather than doing a long series of releases in one session. Experiment with

❖ Too Tight, Too Loose

Although a tight psoas is the more common complaint, habits such as thrusting the hips forward or standing with the lower rib cage poking out can overstretch both the abdominal muscles and the upper fibers of the psoas. Wearing high heels can radically tip the pelvis and rib cage forward. Lack of integrity in these structures decreases their ability to support and stabilize the spine. It's not unusual to encounter people with both conditions: tightness in the lower fibers of the psoas (from slouching and sitting for long periods) *and* looseness in the upper fibers of the psoas. Both conditions lead to dysfunctional movement and almost always result in back pain. ❖

practicing these releasing techniques at the beginning of a routine, in the middle, and at the end. Different sequencing can reap different results. If your sacroiliac joints are unstable, it's best to follow psoas releases with a stabilizing pose such as Bridge Pose (*Setu Bandhasana*; see page 125.)

PRACTICES

Lengthening the Psoas

Benefits
- Gently releases the psoas.
- Builds a stronger felt awareness of the psoas muscles.
- Stabilizes the spine during movement.

Contraindications
- People with pelvic or sacroiliac joint instability should use caution. If gentle asymmetrical lengthening of the psoas creates pain, during or after this inquiry, skip this exercise.
- During the assisted exercise, be careful not to pull too strongly on your partner.

You'll Need
- A yoga mat and blanket.
- A thin washcloth.

Why: Before you can activate a muscle you have to be able to feel it. This inquiry can be invaluable for isolating the specific location and sensation of the psoas.

How

Variation A—Lengthening the Psoas: Lie in CRP. Fold a thin washcloth so that it is 5 centimeters (2 inches) wide and about 1-1/4 centimeters (1/2 inch) thick or fold a yoga belt in half. Place the washcloth or yoga belt under T12 (just above the waist at the base of the rib cage). Step your feet closer to your buttocks. Now place your hands softly at the psoas attachments on the right side. Bring your awareness to the origin of the psoas and gently anchor the spine downward, touching the washcloth or yoga belt. Maintaining contact with the prop, as you exhale, lengthen the right psoas by projecting the knee over the ankle. Track the knee directly over the ankle and foot (you may need to peek down your body to check that the knee is not moving out to the side). This movement will lengthen the insertion of the psoas at the hip away from the origin at the spine (Figure 15A). Keep the movement small to ensure that as you project the knee over the ankle that you do not lift T12 off the floor. Return to neutral on your

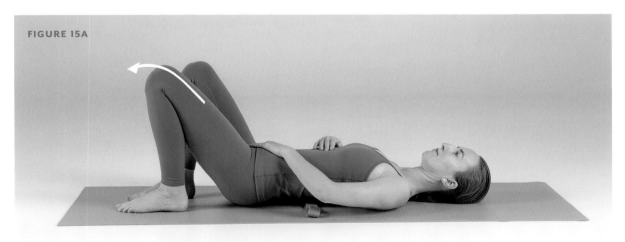

FIGURE 15A

inhalation. Visualize the two attachments moving apart as the psoas lengthens and moving together as you return to the starting position. Repeat several times on the right side, then on the left side, and then alternating sides.

Variation B—Lengthening the Psoas with Pelvis Lifted: Begin in CRP with the knees bent and the feet close to the buttocks. Now lift the pelvis off the floor keeping the pubic bone slightly higher than the navel. On each exhalation, lengthen the right psoas by projecting the right knee over the ankle in the same way as you did in Variation A (Figure 15B). Return to neutral on your inhalation (Figure 15C). Repeat several times on the right side and then on the left side. Then alternate right and left sides an equal number of times. Slowly bring the pelvis back down onto the floor and rest.

Variation C—Lengthening the Psoas with a Partner: For many people, this assisted variation clearly "colors" the psoas in their awareness. Practice this variation on both sides, first with the pelvis on the floor and then with the pelvis off the floor. Your partner will hold the thigh just above the knee and gently draw the thigh away from the pelvis to encourage the psoas to lengthen (Figure 15D). It can be helpful to do this movement on an extended exhalation. As your partner gently pulls on the top of the thigh, consciously anchor T12 against the floor and allow the psoas to be passively lengthened. Draw away the thigh for about 30 seconds and then release the thigh. Practice three times on the right side. Pause and notice whether you feel any difference between the two sides and then practice the movement for three times on the left side.

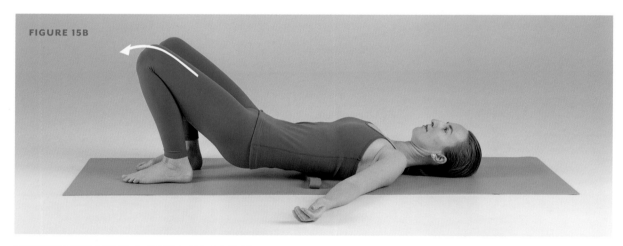

FIGURE 15B

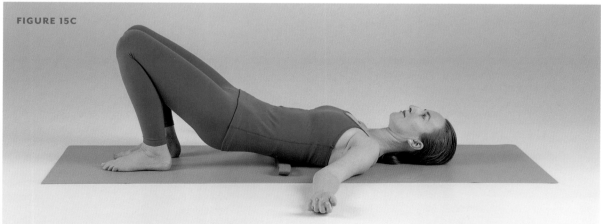

FIGURE 15C

If the psoas is reluctant to release, you can trick it into lengthening by first contracting it. As you inhale, contract the psoas by gently trying to pull your knee toward your chest against the resistance of your partner's hands. On the exhalation, release the contraction and allow your partner to gently lengthen the psoas.

Now lift the pelvis slightly off the floor. Continue to anchor T12 against the floor as your partner draws the thigh away from the pelvis (Figure 15E). Practice for three repetitions on each side, bringing your pelvis onto the floor between releases. Finish by resting for a few minutes in CRP. Finally, extend your legs along the floor.

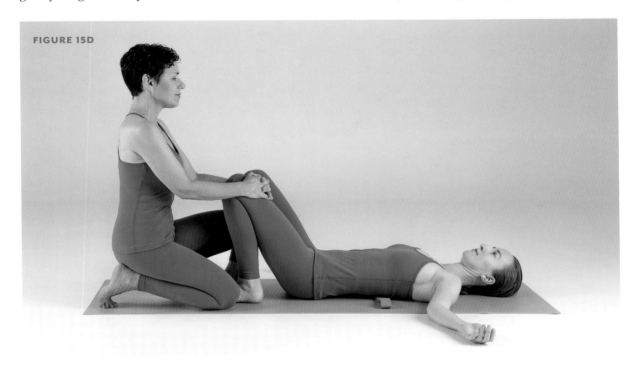

FIGURE 15D

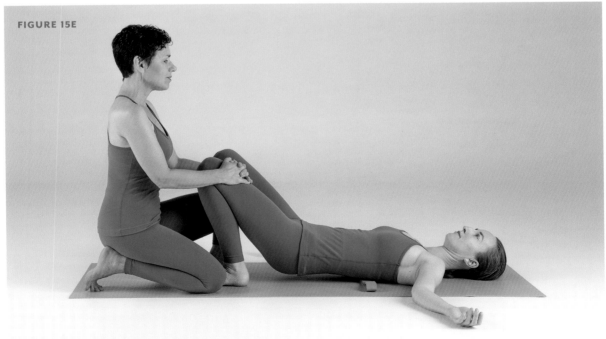

FIGURE 15E

Notice how your body is lying on the floor. Do you feel more or less curvature in the lumbar spine? Does the spine feel longer? Is more of your body in contact with the floor?

Half Bow (*Ardha Dhanurasana*) with Isometric Release

Benefits
- Top pick for releasing a tight and constricted psoas.
- Creates incredible length and release to the groin and helps to lengthen the lower back.
- Helps to release a compressed sacroiliac joint.
- May relieve sciatica.

Contraindications
- People with spondylolysis, spondylolisthesis, or spinal stenosis should use caution. In mild cases of these conditions, a cushion or folded blanket placed between the groins and ribs will support the spine so this practice can be done safely.
- Pregnancy or recent abdominal surgery.

You'll Need
- A yoga mat and blanket.
- Muscle Release Ball (MR Ball); if you don't have an MR Ball, you can still do this practice without it.[2]

Why: When the psoas is in lockdown mode, any attempts to stretch it can result in even greater defensive shortening of the muscle. When a muscle is actively contracted, however, relaxation follows. By asking the psoas to contract, we trick it into releasing. This practice is extremely effective.

How: Lying prone on your cushioned yoga mat, place a half-deflated MR Ball under the right groin, so that the inside edge touches the midline of the pubic bone, and the bulk of the ball fills the groin space. Bend the right knee and ankle 90 degrees so the sole of the foot is flat to the ceiling. Begin by gently pressing the right knee into the floor on an inhalation for 7 seconds (Figure 16A). You need not press forcefully—only make 20 percent of your normal effort. Keeping the foot flexed, lift the knee off the floor on an exhalation for 3–5 seconds (Figure 16B). Raise your knee until you feel a gentle stretch in the anterior thigh and groin. In rhythm with the breath, alternate pressing the knee into the floor isometrically and then lift it off the floor.[3] As you lift, be careful not to externally rotate the leg. You can avoid this rotation by keeping the sole of the foot facing the ceiling. Repeat for five to seven rounds and then remove the MR Ball and lie prone for a few moments. Then roll over on your back and lie supine with your legs extended. Observe whether you feel any difference between the two sides. Now repeat on the left side.

This exercise can result in significant changes in the length of the psoas muscle. However, if the upper fibers of your psoas are very tight, it's likely that you will tend to bend exclusively between T12 and the upper lumbar when you lift the knee off the floor. To stabilize the origin of the psoas, experiment with placing the hands under your forehead and slightly pressing the sternum *away* from the floor as you lift the leg. This will reduce the curvature in the thoracolumbar region and help to target the release of the psoas. You can also experiment with sliding the knee away from the body before you lift it off the floor. This lengthens the psoas and reduces the tendency to hinge at T12.

Half Bow Variation with a Towel: After several days (or weeks) of practicing the primary variation, you may wish to try placing a folded towel or blanket under your bent knee (Figure 16C).

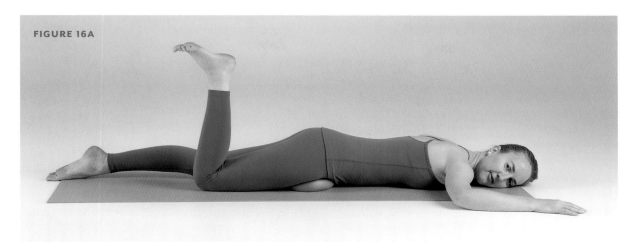

FIGURE 16A

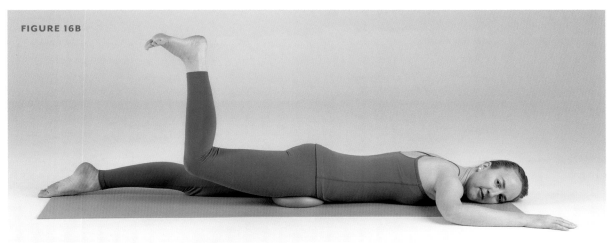

FIGURE 16B

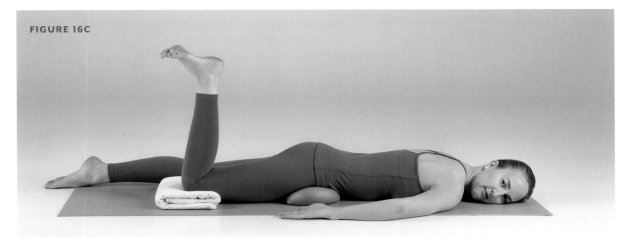

FIGURE 16C

This will increase the resting length of the psoas. Practice alternating pressing your knee downward into the towel (with just 20 percent of your normal effort) and then lifting it off the towel. As your psoas gradually lengthens over time, you can increase the thickness of the folded towel or blanket.

High Lunge at the Wall (or with a Chair)

Benefits

- Targets the deep insertion points of the psoas and iliacus.
- Creates a deep release for the groin while keeping the lumbar spine in a neutral position.

Contraindications

- Those with groin injuries should avoid this practice.

You'll Need

- A yoga mat and wall.
- A chair if you have a tight groin.

Why: Almost any lunge position will open the psoas muscles to some degree. However, if like many people, you have weak core muscles (and a tight psoas), it's likely that when you practice a lunge position, you simply tip your pelvis forward (anterior tilt), relax your abdominal muscles, and deepen your lumbar curve. Bringing the leg up high on the wall (or chair) creates a slight posterior tilt to the pelvis. This helps to keep the pelvis in a neutral position so you can open the psoas without compromising your lower back.

How: Stand close to a wall with your feet hip-width apart. Bend your right knee and bring the

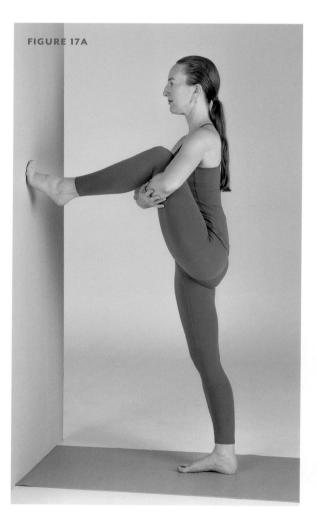

FIGURE 17A

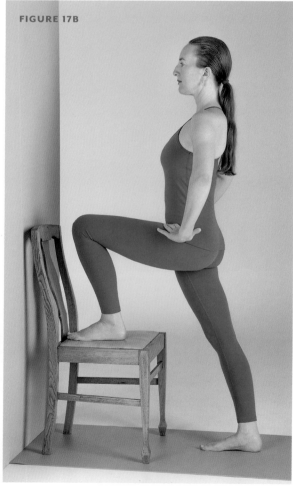

FIGURE 17B

ball of the right foot up as high as you can on the wall (Figure 17A). Wrap your arms around your right thigh and interlock your fingers; maintaining an erect position with your chest. Pressing the ball of your foot into the wall, lift the heel upward. This action has the clever effect of lower-

ing the femur within the hip socket. Maintaining this position, lean slightly toward the wall. If you have limited mobility, simply bring your foot onto the seat of a chair (Figure 17B). Stay for 1 minute, and then release and practice on the other side.

Releasing the Psoas on a Bolster

Benefits
- Elongates the whole of the iliopsoas complex.
- Minimizes strain to the lumbar spine while optimizing deep core release.

Contraindications
- Those with hyperlordosis should be careful not to place the pelvis too far over the bolster (toward the feet), which would only accentuate the lumbar curve.

You'll Need
- A yoga mat and blanket.
- A bolster.

Why: Many people with poor abdominal tone combined with restriction in the psoas muscles fail to release the psoas in a *standing* lunge because the pelvis automatically tips forward (anteriorly) and the lumbar curve becomes more accentuated.

This supine lunge with one leg flexed helps to fix the position of the pelvis so that the extension of the other leg can effectively target psoas restriction and simultaneously minimize strain to the lower back.

How: Lie in a supine position with the knees bent. Lift the pelvis off the floor and place a bolster under the pelvis so the sacrum is supported. If you are small or are working with a bolster of a large diameter, you may need to raise the pelvis on several folded blankets (or use a skinnier bolster). Note that the higher your support, the more challenging it is to release the psoas without compromising the lumbar spine. Begin with both knees bent. Slowly extend your right leg along the floor as you draw the left knee in toward your chest (Figure 18A). Shift your position on the bolster toward your head if you feel discomfort in

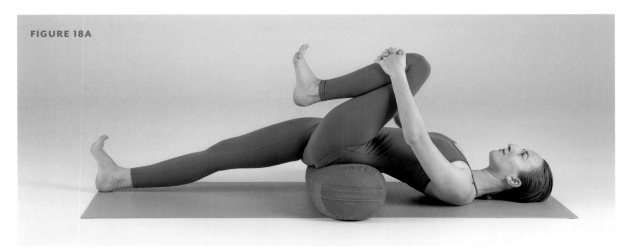

FIGURE 18A

your lower back. If your right knee bends in this position, you can place a support under your heel until the leg is straight. If you feel little or nothing in your groin and thigh, experiment with moving your pelvis on the bolster toward your feet until you find the right pivot point. Strongly extend through the right foot as you lengthen through the whole of the back body. Imagine that your right leg begins from the top of the right kidney and extends all the way to the heel.[4] A slight internal rotation of your right leg will help release the psoas. Stay in this release position for 1 minute. You can create an oscillatory lengthening movement by extending through the right heel as you inhale and pointing the toes as you exhale. Take a few moments to feel the difference between the two sides and then try the movement on the left side.

Thunderbolt Variation with a Partner: This Thunderbolt variation is exceptional for targeting psoas tightness both at the groin and along the length of the muscle. We find that students with chronic lumbar compression love this assisted release as it gives them immediate relief.

Lie on your back with the right leg extended and the left knee drawn in toward your chest. If your psoas is very tight, you will have a large gap between the back of the right thigh and the floor. Your partner can now assist you by kneeling next to your right thigh and pressing down with their hand on the top of the thigh close to the groin. A slight inward rotation of the thigh will help to stabilize the insertion of the iliopsoas (Figure 18B). Let your partner know how much pressure feels comfortable and be clear about asking them to ease off.[5] As you exhale, you may be able to receive more pressure, and as you inhale, it may feel nice to have your partner slightly release the pressure. Work in this way with your breath, staying for at least 1 minute. Then practice the release on the other side.

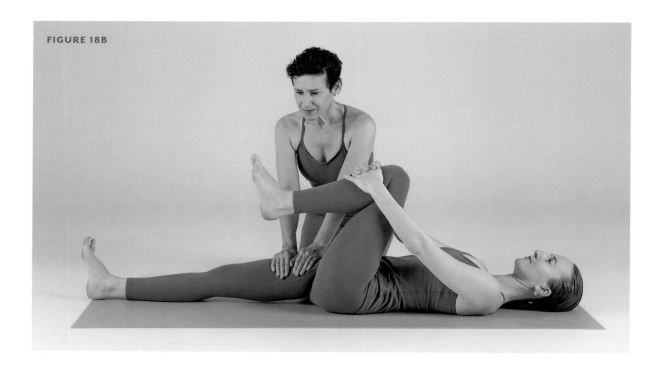

FIGURE 18B

Cobra Pose (*Bhujangasana*)

Benefits

- Contributes to the health of spinal disks.
- Increases flexibility and strength of the spine.
- Opens the chest.
- Lengthens the psoas muscles in a safe way.

Contraindications

- Spondylolysis, spondylolisthesis, or severe spinal stenosis.
- Pregnancy, recent abdominal surgery, or wrist injury.
- People with hyperlordosis should be cautious and do only a small movement, preferably with more support under the belly.

You'll Need

- A yoga mat and one or two blankets.
- A bolster for the variation.

Why: Cobra Pose can cause discomfort when practiced in a way that compresses the curves in the neck and low back. In this variation, the psoas muscles are consciously lengthened so the lumbar spine remains long and decompressed throughout the posture. The use of blankets or a bolster supports the pelvis and lower lumbar spine and helps to prevent hinging in the vulnerable vertebrae where the spine transitions from areas of greater movement to areas of less movement (between L1 and the rib cage and L5 and the sacrum). When the movement is visualized as a lengthening of the psoas in the middle of the body, the tendency to compress the lumbar curve is reduced. Lowering your gaze and maintaining the length in your neck also assists in reducing compression in the lower back.

How: In the classic practice of Cobra Pose, the hands are placed under the shoulders and the head and neck are extended backward. Both of these practices dramatically increase the compression into the neck and lumbar spine. In the following variations, we have altered the position of the arms and neck to minimize stress to the spine. Begin with Variation A with your lower abdomen supported on folded blankets. If you feel comfortable in Variation A, you may wish to try the more advanced work in Variation B. If you feel compression in your lower back in Variation A, try Variation C with your abdomen supported on a bolster.

Variation A—Cobra Pose with Blankets: Place two folded blankets across your yoga mat. Lie on the blankets so that your lower abdomen is resting on the edge of the blanket and your thighs are resting on the mat. Place your elbows shoulder-width apart and slightly in front of your shoulders with the forearms turned out 20–30 degrees. Feel the two most prominent points of the left and right pelvic crests; press these points firmly into the blanket to activate your core muscles. On an exhalation, raise your upper body slightly off the floor, elongating the spine and psoas muscles as you anchor the groin (Figure 19A). This movement takes place in the middle of the body from the groin to the solar plexus. Visualize the psoas lifting the front of the spine so the back muscles don't have to work so hard. The elbows and forearms are simply supporting the movement of the spine. Press the sternum back into the body to stabilize the spinal insertion point. This will help to prevent excessive extension at the vulnerable juncture point between the base of the thoracic spine (bottom of the rib cage) and the top of the lumbar spine (L1) (Figure 19B, incorrect). Relax slightly as you inhale and attempt to come a little higher on your exhalation, moving your hands back toward your shoulders if you can do so without discomfort. Stay for three to five breaths and repeat three times.

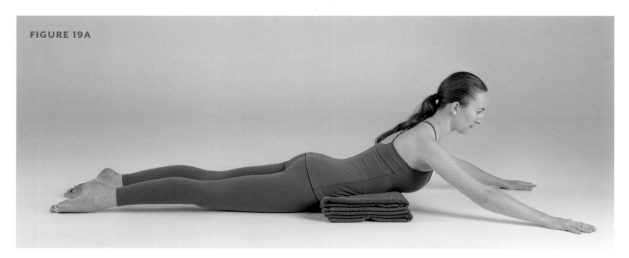

FIGURE 19A

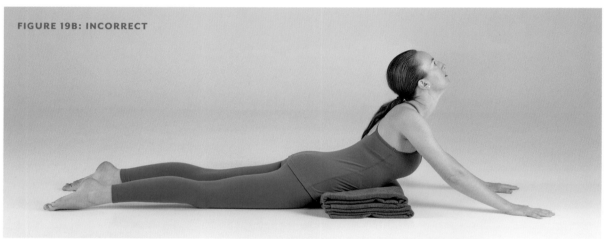

FIGURE 19B: INCORRECT

If you feel any compression or discomfort in your lower back when you raise your body away from the floor, slide your hands farther away from your body. This will decrease the degree of extension (Figure 19C). Ensure that the neck remains elongated and your gaze low, which also will reduce the extension in your lower back. If after modifying your position you still feel discomfort in your lower back, immediately release back into Child's Pose (*Balasana*, see Figure 19D). Child's Pose is a simple way to release your back and can be practiced in between each stay in Cobra Pose or at the end of several repetitions.

Variation B—Cobra Pose with One Bent Knee: You can also experiment by bending one knee and then the other while holding the Cobra Pose (Fig-

ure 19E). Flex the foot as you do this and notice whether the extension of the thigh deepens the release of the psoas on that side.

Variation C—Cobra Pose with a Bolster: This variation of Cobra Pose never fails to bring a smile to those who have never managed to practice the classical versions of Cobra Pose without discomfort in their lower backs. It's simple. Place a bolster along the length of your yoga mat and lie with your pubic bone right on the back edge of the bolster with your pelvis supported. Place your arms on either side of the bolster (as in Variation A). Slowly lift your elbows off the floor, sliding the hands farther out if you need to reduce the degree of extension in your back. Anchor your groin (the insertion of the psoas muscles) on

FIGURE 19C

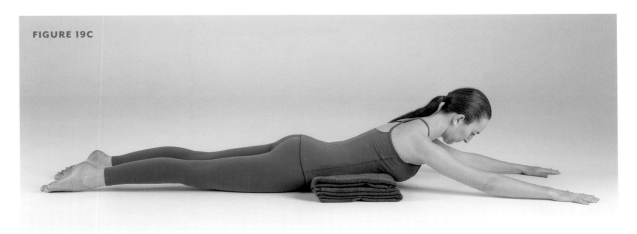

FIGURE 19D

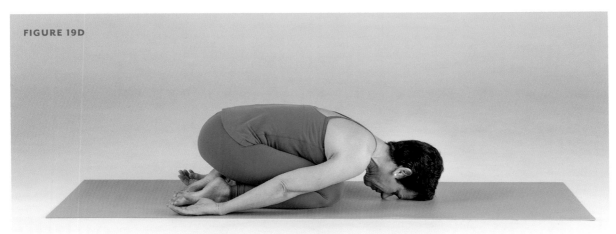

FIGURE 19E

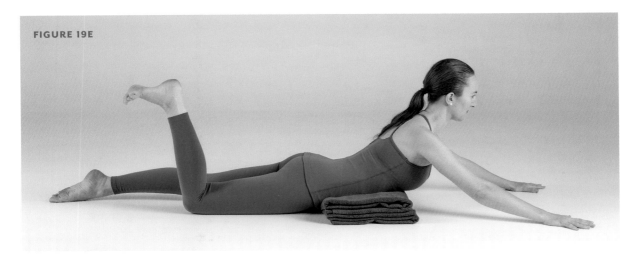

the edge of the bolster as you elongate the spine forward and up (Figure 19F). Surprised? Raising your pelvis on the bolster has changed the relationship between your spine, pelvis, and legs, radically reducing the degree of resting exten-sion in your lumbar spine. This distributes the extension over a greater length of your spine. You may want to practice this variation for some time before attempting Cobra Pose with the pelvis on the floor.

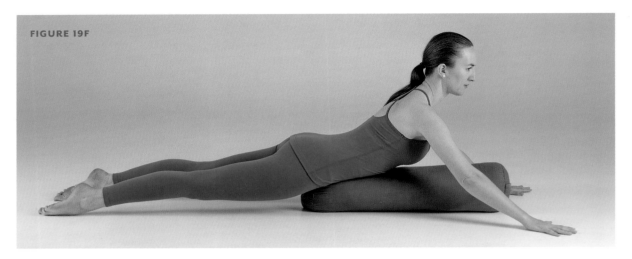

FIGURE 19F

If you find yourself in a Yoga class where Upward Facing Dog (*Urdhva Mukha Svanasana*) is a practiced during the Sun Salutation (*Suryanamaskar*), and that practice consistently irritates your back, consider practicing Cobra Pose with the bolster instead. Let your teacher know that you need to modify your practice to heal your spine. If your teacher is not sympathetic of your need to make this modification, it may be time to find a new teacher!

Therapeutic Psoas Release

Benefits
- Lengthens and releases the spinal and psoas muscles.
- Helps to decompress the sacroiliac joint.
- Calms and steadies the nervous system.

Contraindications
- People with disc problems should be cautious. If you feel any discomfort, this practice is not suitable for you at this time.
- Those with varicosities (varicose veins) should not place weight on the lower legs.

You'll Need
- A yoga mat and a bolster.
- A chair.
- Two or three blankets.
- A partner.

Why: Remember how our evolution from quadruped to biped changed the relationship of the psoas to gravity? In Chapter Two, we noted that people with acute back pain often are reduced to crawling on all-fours. In this position, we place the legs in an upside-down all-fours position. This gently compresses the psoas and paradoxically helps it to release.

How: Place a folded blanket on the seat of the chair to cushion the surface and hard edges. Cushion your yoga mat with another blanket and lie down with your torso on the floor, with your lower legs resting on the seat of the chair. Alternatively, use your living room couch (it is often the perfect height for this practice). Ensure that your heels are supported and that your lower legs are parallel to the ground. If your heels are hanging in space, this will put strain on your lower back. If so, you may need to raise your torso by putting two folded blankets under your trunk. Now experiment with the angle between your

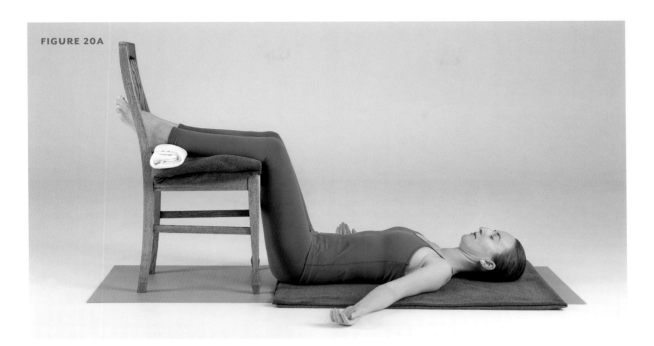

FIGURE 20A

thigh and your pelvis by moving closer to or far-ther away from the chair. You are searching for the point at which your femurs relax into the hip sockets and the psoas and spinal muscles soften (Figure 20A). Stay in this pose for 5–15 minutes.

Therapeutic Psoas Release Variation with Weight: The addition of weight on your shins can make a phenomenal difference to the degree of decompression you experience in your sacro-iliac joint and lower lumbar spine. It's not easy, however, to manipulate a heavy bolster onto your lower legs by yourself without putting your back in a vulnerable position. Ask a friend to place the bolster across your lower legs. Then stand-ing behind the chair facing your head, have your friend gradually increase the weight by pressing downward on the bolster with both hands (Figure 20B). If this feels wonderful and your friend is not too heavy, have them sit on the bolster itself (Fig-ure 20C). This variation is not for everyone, but we have found that students with the most debil-itating back pain often receive powerful results from this practice. Like any powerful medicine, use it cautiously, and be sure to have your friend

remove the bolster before you come out of the posture. Stay for up to 5 minutes with the weight on the shins. To come out of the pose, gently lower your legs to the floor and relax in CRP or with the legs extended.

PRACTICE SUMMARY

- Lengthening the Psoas Variations A, B, and C
- Half Bow with Isometric Release
- High Lunge at the Wall (or with a Chair)
- Releasing the Psoas on a Bolster
- Thunderbolt Variation with a Partner
- Cobra Pose Variations A, B, and C
- Child's Pose
- Therapeutic Psoas Release

Rather than doing all of these releases in one ses-sion, use this summary to tweak your memory of these practices. We recommend that you learn each release individually and then incorporate up to three practices in your routine. For instance, you might do the High Lunge at the Wall just before you practice standing postures, or the Half Bow with Isometric Release before the practice of

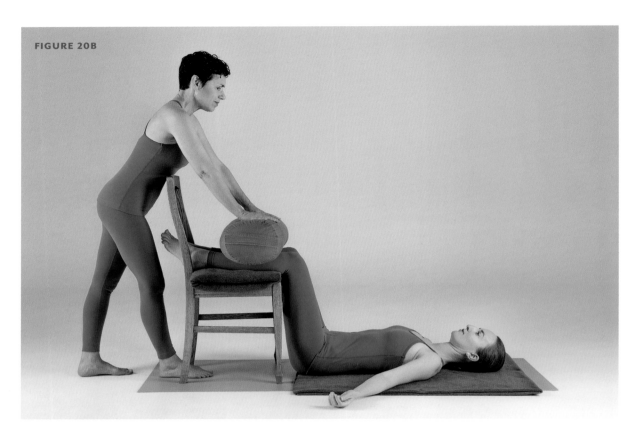

FIGURE 20B

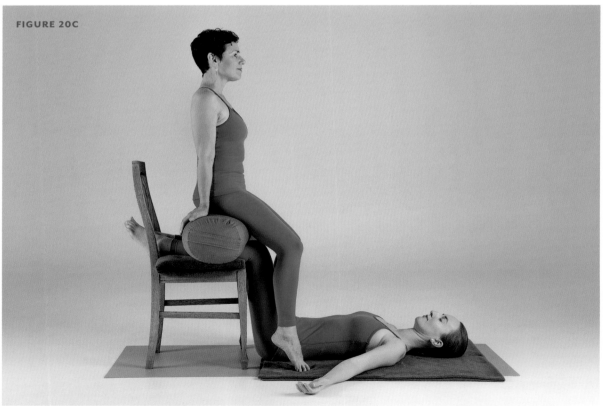

FIGURE 20C

more traditional back bends, such as Bow Pose (*Dhanurasana*). Thunderbolt can be fantastic as a counter pose after standing work toward the end of a practice. And the Therapeutic Psoas Release using a chair can be an alternative to Corpse Pose (*Savasana*). All of the practices in this section are designed to increase your somatic intelligence and help you to be more conscious of initiating both hip and lumbar extension from the deep psoas muscles. Once you have practiced these movements, we encourage you to carry your newfound learning into your movement, Yoga practice, sports activities, and tasks of daily living.

After practicing each technique take a little time to observe any changes. Lie on your back with your legs extended straight. Are you more comfortable? Is more of your body on the floor? Have the spinal curves altered? Go for a stroll. Does your back feel more upright as you walk? If you proceed to practice other Yoga postures, is strain reduced in your lower back, and can you feel new sensations in previously hard-to-reach spots like the upper back, groin, or shoulders?

Having long, strong, and pliant core muscles means you can move with the least amount of effort and that your limbs can coordinate around a mobile center. Notice how the restoration of this long central axis in the body allows the other more superficial muscles of the body to relax. Feel, too, how this deepening sense of connection between your plumb line and gravity creates a grounded verticality. As you stand in your own center of gravity, notice how this affects your state of mind, the harmony of your emotions, and the skillfulness with which you move through the world.

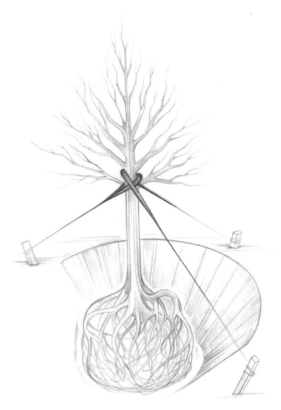

ILLUSTRATION 21: Psoas Muscles of Equal Length Act Like Guy-Wires to Promote Straightness of the Spine.

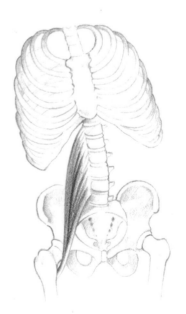

ILLUSTRATION 22A: Unilateral Tightness of Psoas

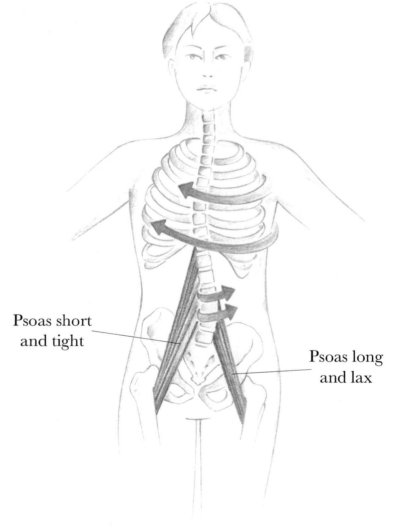

Psoas short and tight

Psoas long and lax

ILLUSTRATION 22B: Secondary Compensations of Unilateral Psoas Tightness

CHAPTER 6

Balance

L ET'S RETURN TO our image of the sapling tree being supported by guy-wires to ensure that the tree grows straight and tall. Imagine if one of those supporting ropes was shorter than the others. Undoubtedly, the tree would begin to tilt and veer off an ideal vertical axis until some observant gardener adjusted the tension between the guy-wires (Illustration 21). This analogy, however, only goes so far in that the pelvis, sacroiliac joints, and lumbar spine (and everything else above and below these structures), represent an infinitely more complex mechanical structure.

Two concepts will help us to understand the mechanics of spinal imbalance: (1) when the spine bends to one side (lateral flexion), it also induces rotation of the vertebral segments; and (2) when the spine twists (rotates) this action is always accompanied by some degree of lateral flexion. Thus, any unilateral pull on the spine, whether from the psoas or other muscles, has the potential to cause complex rotations, lateral deviations, and a cascade of compensations in the structures above and below. This is especially true for anyone who has structural scoliosis; a lateral curvature in one part of the spine may be compensated by a secondary curvature (or curvatures) in other parts of the vertebral column.[1] These compensations are almost always the body's attempt to find a midline point that will bring the eyes in line with the horizon.

Contemporary research tells us that the psoas is designed primarily to be a *stabilizer* of the spine rather than a *mover* of the spine. Yet paradoxically, any chronic shortening and hardening of the psoas can have a huge impact on spinal alignment. When one side of the psoas becomes shorter than the other, this can cause the spine to side bend, followed by compensations such as spinal and rib cage rotation, hip hiking, and sacroiliac dysfunction (Illustrations 22A and 22B). Not surprisingly, unilateral contraction of the psoas almost always involves the neighboring muscle quadratus lumborum (or QL as it is commonly known). Remember that QL originates from the posterior crest of the ilium and inserts onto the 12th rib and the transverse processes of the 1st–4th lumbar vertebrae (Illustration 23A). When the pelvis is

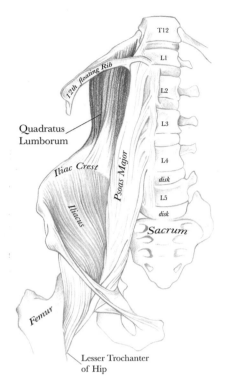

Quadratus Lumborum

ILLUSTRATION 23A

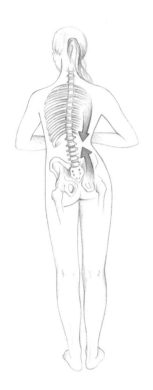

Unilateral Tightness of Quadratus Lumborum

ILLUSTRATION 23B

fixed, contraction of QL on one side causes side bending of the lumbar spine and rib cage. When the ribs and spine are fixed, it can hike up the pelvis on one side (Illustration 23B). Thus, QL has the capacity to trigger imbalance in the psoas, and vice versa. Although many clinical causes can contribute to one-sided spinal discomfort, when muscle shortening is significant on one side of the lumbar spine, there's a strong likelihood that QL and the psoas are in cahoots, creating havoc!

WORKING TOWARD SYMMETRY

Our experience working with students who have long-standing asymmetrical challenges in their bodies has shown that focusing on the minutia of these rotations and counter-rotations can be frustrating and counterproductive. In some cases, perfect symmetry simply is not possible,

especially with some congenital defects. Rather than becoming obsessed with obtaining a perfect symmetry, it can be far more productive to focus on improving function. With regular and careful practice, however, little adjustments *toward symmetry* can make a *big* difference to function. Even a few millimeters of newly created space over the span of the lower back can take pressure off of facet joints, reduce inflammation, increase movement capacity, and even lead to complete amelioration of pain. The desire to be pain free and to maintain the ability to move with ease can be a strong motivation to sustain self-care regimens. We have seen many students with significant structural challenges, and many who have sustained serious injuries (for which they have been given a poor prognosis), regain exceptional function. Furthermore, we also work with students who have symmetrical bodies but through poor posture and lack of integrated movement, have less adeptness and movement function than those with structural challenges who maintain regular self-care regimens.

We use a simple approach when we identify a one-sided "snag" in the psoas and QL:

1. Elongate (a bent wire becomes straighter as it is pulled on each end).

2. Laterally extend (the shortened side is lengthened, and the overstretched side is strengthened).

3. Derotate (a natural consequence of the first two steps).

Before you begin these exercises, take a few moments to assess your body balance. Doing so will help you to notice and appreciate changes when they do occur. If you are a teacher or somatic practitioner, guiding your clients through a brief body scan can help them to identify imbalances and also maintain new postural habits.

In addition to the inquiries and psoas tests that follow, it can be valuable to stand unclothed in front of a full-length mirror. Are the shoulders even? Are the two sides of the waist the same or is one more indented than the other? Unevenness in one or both of these two areas is a clear indication that a lateral imbalance exists in the body.

⠿ INQUIRIES: *Assessing Body Balance*

Benefits
- Establishes your starting point.
- Develops awareness of asymmetries and structural imbalances.

Contraindications
- None.

You'll Need
- A yoga mat.
- A bolster or folded blanket.

Why: Your structural imbalances often feel "normal" because the compensations dictated by your nervous system have become unconscious habitual patterns. As you learn to sense and feel differences between the two sides of your body, you can begin to address these imbalances. For instance, if one hip is noticeably more restricted or if you feel persistent tension on one side of your lower back, these are clues that may indicate psoas imbalance. In the following inquiries, you will be asked to assume various positions and movements to determine whether you can

identify differences in the symmetry and function of the two sides of your body. Your findings will set a base level so that after practicing any of the inquiries or exercises in this book, you can make more accurate assessments of the changes that have occurred. You also will have a better idea of which side needs greater release or engagement.

How: Start in a simple standing position on a level surface. Close your eyes and deliberately withdraw your attention from the outer world and turn it inward. Take a few calming breaths to slow your mind. Make an intention to simply notice any body imbalances in a nonjudgmental way and without any need to change your experience. An attitude of "Oh, isn't that interesting!" is much more helpful than "I'm so imbalanced!" Take your time and spend several breaths noticing the sensations in each part of the body you are scanning. ⠿

:: Standing Body Scan

Feet: Direct your attention to the contact between your feet and the ground. Are the feet bearing weight equally? Is one foot pressing more heavily or lifting away from the ground? Do the arches feel equally raised? When you look down at your feet, are both feet pointing straight ahead or does one foot rotate outward more than the other?

Knees: Move your attention to the knees. Is your body weight transferred through the middle of the knee joints or off-center in one or both legs? Are both knees equally extended or is one more flexed or extended than the other?

Hips: Move your attention to the femoral joints. Does the weight of the pelvis feel balanced on the femoral heads or is one side of the pelvis sitting more heavily on one hip than the other? Is one hip more forward than the other?

Lower Back: Turn your attention to the low back and pelvis. Is there more tension on one side of the lower back?

Balancing: Stand on one foot for two to three breaths. Repeat on the other side. Is it easier to balance on one side? Does one side feel stronger? Does your pelvis shift laterally (out to the side)

more on one leg than the other? Now stand on one foot with the hands clasped behind the head. Draw up the opposite knee as if you were marching until it is higher than the hip (Figure 21). Can you hold it for 5 seconds? Repeat on the other side. ::

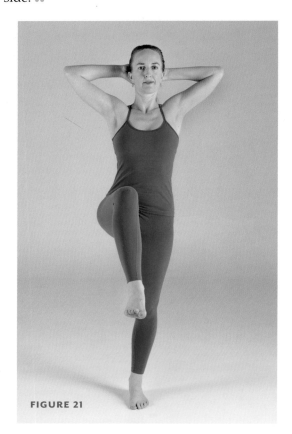

FIGURE 21

:: Supine Body Scan

Lie in a supine position with both legs straight. If this position is uncomfortable, place a bolster under your knees.

Points of Contact: Notice how your body weight rests into the ground. Is one side of the body resting more heavily against the ground than the other?

Feet: Move your attention to your feet and notice whether one heel feels heavier than the other. When you look down at your feet, is one more externally rotated than the other?

Knees: Move your attention to your knees. Is the back of the knee closer to the floor on one side?

Sacrum: Notice your sacrum. Is one side pressing into the floor more than the other?

Spine: Notice your spine. Is the space between the floor and lumbar spine the same on both sides? Is the sensation in the muscles along the length of your spine similar on both sides? ⠿

⠿ Assessing Your Psoas

Test 1: If you are uncomfortable when you lie supine with both legs straight, skip this first inquiry. Place your hands palms down and fingertips touching in the hollow between your lower back and the floor. This will help you monitor any movement of the lumbar spine as you move your legs. Slowly drag one heel toward the pelvis and notice whether the lumbar spine stays neutral or slightly flexes toward the floor or whether it arches and moves away from the floor on that

side (Figure 22A, correct; Figure 22B, incorrect). Repeat on the other side. Finally, repeat the flexion movement drawing both heels into the pelvis at the same time. If the lumbar spine arches or the ribs poke out, the psoas is not strong enough to stabilize the spine.

Test 2: Bend both knees and lift the pelvis off the floor. Place one or two blankets or a bolster under the pelvis so that the sacrum is supported. Bend

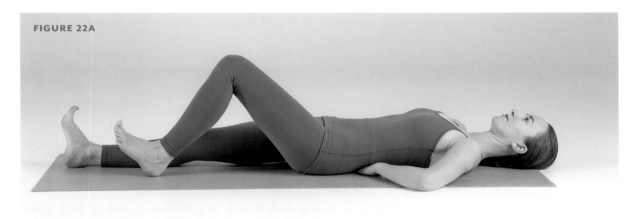

FIGURE 22A

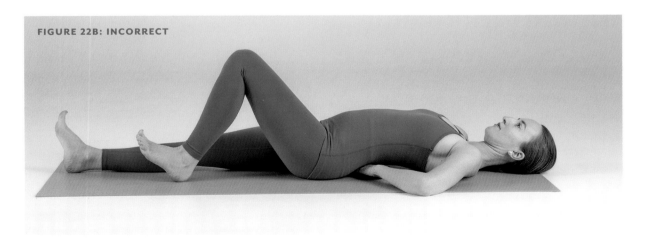

FIGURE 22B: INCORRECT

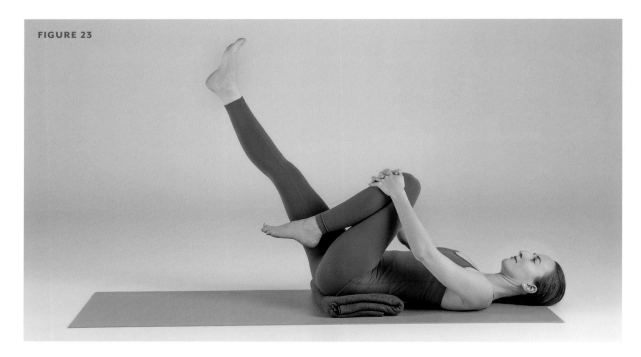

FIGURE 23

both knees into the chest then extend the right leg up toward the ceiling. Slowly lower the straight leg to the floor (Figure 23). How much effort does this movement require? Does the movement cause any discomfort? Does your back arch or do your ribs poke out? Does your leg stay straight throughout the journey to the floor or does the knee bend? Do you tense the back of your neck?

Repeat on the other side and notice any differences. If any of these compensations occur, the psoas may be shortened on one side.

After completing these inquiries, do you have a better sense of which psoas may be in need of more attention?

PRACTICES

Spinal Release on the Chair

Benefits

- Releases and elongates the spine while it is in a neutral and supported position.
- Helps to realign and release asymmetrical imbalances.
- Provides a gentle form of traction.

Contraindications

- People with compromised disk integrity may need to raise the chest slightly higher than the pelvis to ensure that they maintain a neutral lumbar curvature (i.e., the lumbar spine should be slightly indented). If this does not alleviate discomfort, this practice may not be suitable for you at this time.

You'll Need

- Two chairs (with flat rather than tilted seats and a leg on each corner—dining room chairs are ideal).
- Two blankets.
- A bolster or pillow to support the knees.

Why: When spinal muscles have become chronically shortened or imbalanced, it can be extremely beneficial to open the space between the vertebral segments. More active forms of traction do not always feel comfortable, however, especially when muscles are in a state of spasm. Supporting the front of the body with the spine in a neutral position allows the deep muscles of the back to relax and let go.

How

Variation A—Symmetrical Traction: First put a yoga mat underneath your chairs so that they will remain secure. Place a folded blanket on the seat of each chair to cushion the surface. Place a bolster to the side of the first chair and rest your knees on the bolster; then lie belly-down across the seat of the chair with your arms and head resting on the edge of the second chair (Figure 24A). You may need an extra blanket under your head and arms to feel supported, and depending on the length of your legs, you may want to remove the bolster support or use folded blankets instead. Your thighs should feel supported rather than be hanging off the edge of the chair. The whole trunk will be supported completely by the seat of the chair, and the spine should be in a neutral position. Focus on breathing deeply with an emphasis on releasing tension on your exhalation. Relax for 3–5 minutes and then gently come out of the pose.

Variation B—Asymmetrical Traction: For those with asymmetrical changes in the lower back, it can be helpful to reach forward and rest your forehead on the edge of the second chair and extend the arms more actively by taking hold of the back of the chair. If you have distinct tension on one side of your back, begin by shifting the chair a few inches *away* from that side (e.g., shift the chair to the right if you feel tension on the left side of the back; Figure 24B). You may find it helpful to have a friend move the chair for you. Notice whether this shift to one side alleviates or exacerbates the tension in your back. If you are feeling a sense of decompression and relief, stay here for 1 minute or more. Then come back to the centered position and notice whether you still feel discomfort on one side of your back. If you feel immediate discomfort when you move the chair off-center, come back to the centered position. Carefully move the

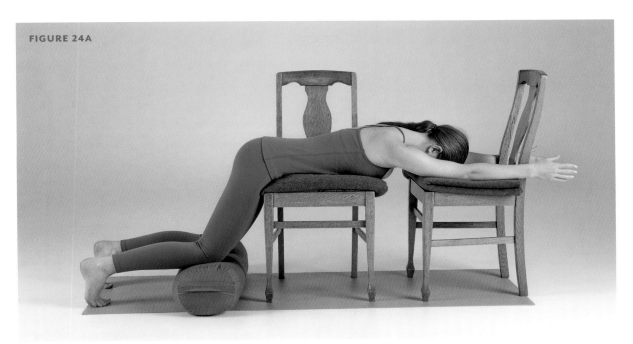

FIGURE 24A

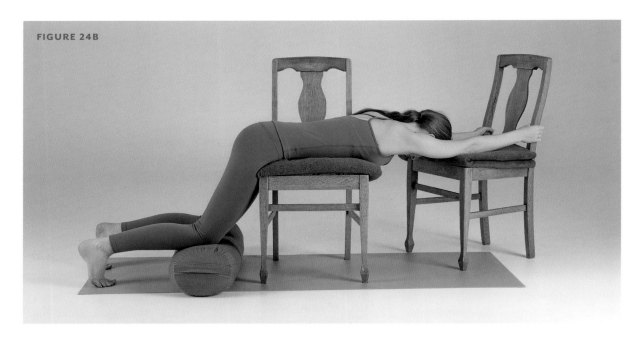

FIGURE 24B

chair a few inches to the left and repeat the experiment. Even if you have distinct shortness on one side of your lower back and waist, it can be helpful to laterally extend to both sides as the complex rotations within the spine will be addressed more effectively by working with both sides. Certainly if a practice causes you pain, don't persist.

Balancing Quadratus Lumborum
This exercise was inspired by the work of Thomas Hanna.[2]

Benefits
- Gently laterally extends and decompresses the lumbar spine.
- Releases chronic tension and helps to balance the two sides of QL.
- Lengthens the intervertebral muscles through the lumbar and lower thoracic spine.
- Counterbalances the spine after practicing movements of extension (back bending) or flexion (forward bending).

Contraindications
- People with compromised disk integrity, prolapsed disks, or spinal stenosis should be cautious especially if twisting currently exacerbates their condition.

You'll Need
- A yoga mat and yoga blanket.

Why: QL is a deep muscle of the posterior abdominal wall. This simple and effective exercise helps to release and balance the two sides of this muscle. Creating symmetry between the two sides can help to realign the lumbar spinal vertebrae. Because unilateral tautness of QL can cause one iliac crest to hike upward, releasing this tension can help to level the pelvis and promote optimal function of the sacroiliac joints.

How: So that you can appreciate the effects of this practice, first sit in a kneeling position on the floor. Shift your hips to the right of your feet. Gently turn the body to the right bringing your left arm to rest on the outside of the right knee and using your right arm to support your spine in a vertical position to assume Sage Pose I (*Bharadvajasana I*: Figure 25A). Notice the sensation in your lower back and also how far you can twist to this side. Then release the twist and slide your right arm along the floor to come into the side-lying position for the QL release (Figure 25B).

Lie on your right side with your right arm extended on the floor over your head. Bend your knees, so that your thighs are at a right angle to your abdomen. Take a moment to check that the back of your head is in line with the back of your pelvis so that you are in a truly side-lying position with the spine in a neutral position. The first time you practice this exercise, it can be helpful to place your back against a wall. You may be surprised how far back the head and chest need to be to accurately align the body in a side-lying position. Keeping the knees together, slowly lift the left lower leg, inhaling as you come up and lowering to a count of four as you exhale (Figure 25C). Practice five to seven times. Notice how the right side of your waist extends toward the floor and the left side shortens. Your right QL will be lengthening as your left QL contracts. Now lift both lower legs together from knee to foot, coming up on an inhalation and lowering to a count of four on an exhalation (Figure 25D). Practice five to seven times.

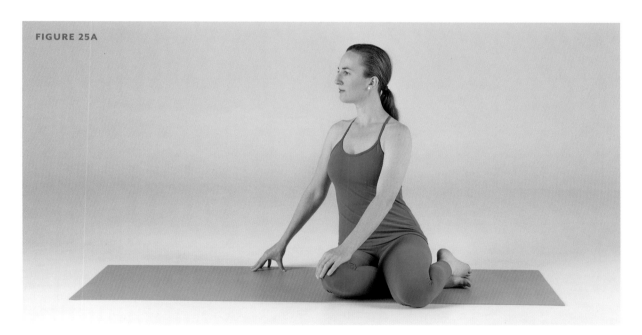

FIGURE 25A

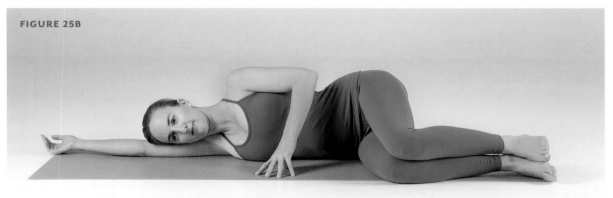

FIGURE 25B

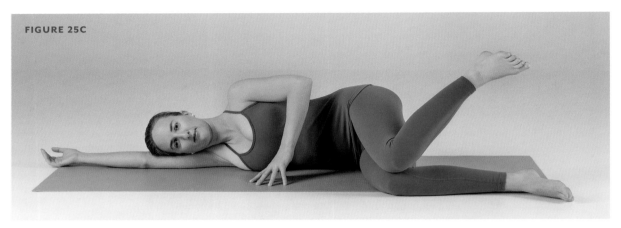

FIGURE 25C

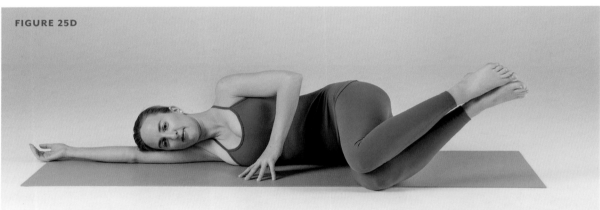

FIGURE 25D

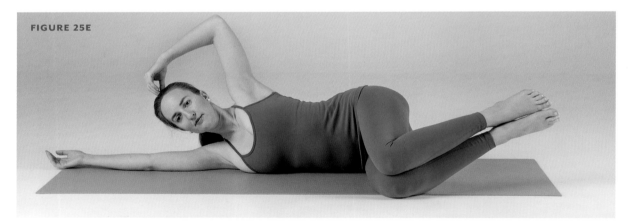

FIGURE 25E

Finally, extend your left arm over your head and touch the crown of the head with your fingertips. Guiding your head with your hand, gently raise the head off the floor. Ensure that your head is not forward of the rest of your body. Do not strain your neck by lifting the head too far (more is not better!). Raise the head on an inhalation and lower it to a count of four on an exhalation.

Practice five to seven times. Now simultaneously raise the head while raising both lower legs (Figure 25E). This variation targets the upper fibers of QL where they attach to the base of the rib cage. And, surprise, surprise, QL's friend and neighbor the psoas is also side bending in all these variations. Practice this movement five to seven times.

Now come back to your seated twist position

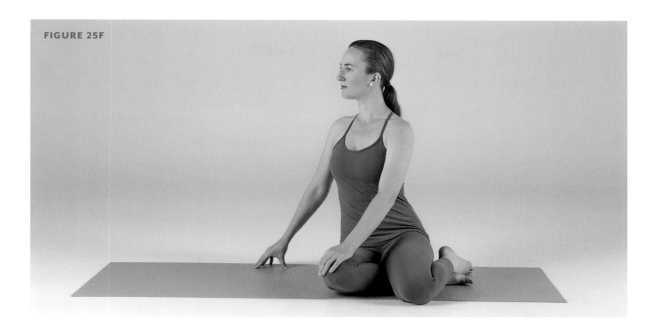

FIGURE 25F

and turn again to the right (Figure 25F). Notice whether you feel any change in the sensation in your lower back. Can you twist to a greater degree and with greater ease? Practice the series on your left side.

If you have a marked difference between the two sides of your waist (e.g., your right side is tighter than your left), we recommend that you practice lengthening the tight side first (i.e., lying on your right side), and then practice lengthening the opposite side (i.e., your left side). You may even wish to repeat the series on your tight side practicing each movement for three repetitions.

Asymmetrical Corpse Pose (*Savasana*)

Benefits
- Helps to release chronic one-sided back tension and discomfort.
- Helps to laterally extend and derotate the lumbar spine.
- Provides relief for people with lumbar scoliosis.

Contraindications
- If you don't need it, don't do it! This asymmetrical variation is only for those with existing spinal imbalances.

You'll Need
- A yoga mat and blanket.
- A bolster or pillow.
- A towel to support the neck and head if you require it.

Why: Because of the fixation on body symmetry in practices such as Yoga, it's not surprising that practicing relaxation in an asymmetrical position rarely occurs to us. If, however, you have an asymmetrical problem in your body, the solution, at least initially, will involve asymmetrical strategies. If you have niggling tension on one side of your back, especially when you lie in relaxation with the legs extended on the floor, you may be delighted to discover how quickly the discomfort abates through the simple action of moving the legs *slightly* off-center. This tiny adjustment can help to open up space in locked lumbar facet joints, reduce compression around nerves (both of which can cause chronic inflammation), and subtly elongate shortened spinal muscles.

How: Lie on a blanketed yoga mat with your legs extended straight. If lying on your back with the legs straight is immediately uncomfortable adjust your position by placing a pillow or bolster under your knees. If you support the knees, ensure that your heels are resting on the floor (or support them with a folded towel). Take a moment to observe the sensation on the right and left sides of your

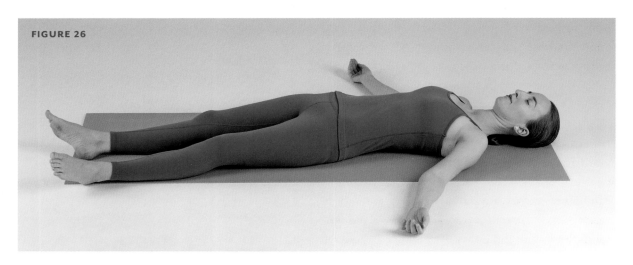

FIGURE 26

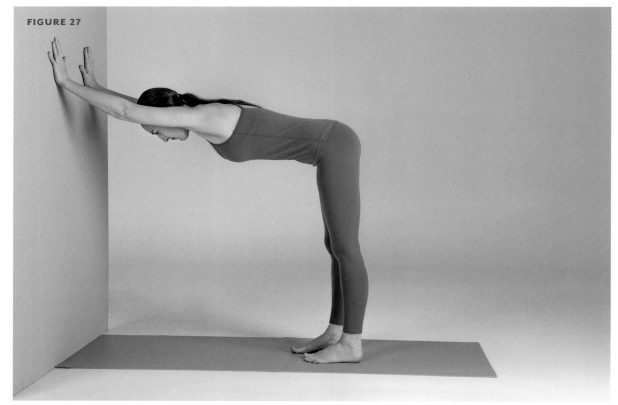

FIGURE 27

lower back. There are no hard and fast rules as to which side to move the legs. Most commonly, if you have discomfort on the right side of the lower back, move your legs several centimeters (an inch or so) off-center to the left (Figure 26).[3] If the tightness and discomfort eases as a result of this maneuver, stay for 3–5 minutes and then return to a symmetrical position. If you feel discomfort when returning to the symmetrical position, bring your legs off-center once again and enjoy your relaxation for another 5–10 minutes.

You can use this strategy in many movements in which the legs otherwise would be symmetrical. In Downward Facing Dog (*Adho Mukha Svanasana*), try placing one foot several centimeters (an inch or more) in front of the other. In Half Downward Facing Dog (*Ardha Adho Mukha Svanasana*) practiced with the hands on a wall, this strategy can be particularly effective if accompanied by a reach of the sitting bones and tail toward the center of the room (Figure 27).

As you go about your day, observe whether you have any "one-sided" habits, such as crossing your legs when you sit. During activities such as gardening, do you always shovel in a particular direction? Could you teach yourself to use both sides of your body when doing household chores such as vacuuming? Learning to do movements evenly on both sides can help to reduce potential overuse and strain and will go a long way toward building functional symmetry in your body.

PRACTICE SUMMARY

- Spinal Release on Chair (Symmetrical Traction)
- Spinal Release on Chair (Asymmetrical Traction)
- Balancing Quadratus Lumborum
- Asymmetrical Corpse Pose

CHAPTER 7

Strength: Activating the Core Cylinder of Support

T O THIS POINT, we have focused on releasing, lengthening, and balancing the psoas muscles as a means to access the deepest level of core support. When the psoas is optimally balanced, the pelvis will be in a centered position and the abdominal organs will rest comfortably inside the pelvic basin. A neutral pelvic position provides an ideal foundation for the spinal column to elongate upward, with balanced spinal curvatures that transition smoothly from one segment of the spine to the next.

CONSCIOUS ACTIVATION OF THE PSOAS MUSCLES

Now, we are ready to consciously contract the psoas and access deep core strength. Once you learn how to engage the psoas, you can visualize it coiling like a spring as it contracts. When a spring compresses, it creates latent power that can give momentum and cohesive strength to the resulting movement. The extensive matrix of fascia that invests the psoas is imbued with viscoelasticity—a quality that supports the dynamic action of coiling and uncoiling that is so important for strength in movement. You may want to refer to the section on viscoelasticity in Chapter Two (see page 31), to refresh your memory.

Learning to consciously switch on the psoas is just as important as learning to soften, lengthen, and balance it. The psoas never works alone in any movement; it contracts in concert with neighboring muscles. Nevertheless, learning to isolate and activate the psoas will help you to initiate movement from the center of the body and enable you to prevent habitual overuse of the superficial duplicators. Remember, the superficial duplicators (the quadriceps and the outer abdominal muscles) can replicate the action of the psoas but with far greater effort. When the psoas is the key initiator of movement, these more superficial muscles can relax into their intended supportive role.

:: INQUIRIES: *Activating Your Psoas*

Lie on your back with the legs straight and the lumbar spine in a neutral position. If this is uncomfortable, place a pillow or bolster under your knees. If you discovered during the previous inquiries that one psoas muscle feels more restricted, then begin your exploration on the less restricted side. Place one hand on the origin and the other hand on the insertion point of the psoas on your chosen side. (You may wish to review Chapter Three, "Tracing the Psoas with Hip Flexion" on page 54). Take a few moments to soften and release the psoas with Abdominal Breathing; a relaxed muscle can contract more efficiently than a tense one.

Choose one of the following images to initiate engagement of the psoas. Experiment with each image to see which one works best for you.

- Envisage the whole muscle condensing, shortening, and widening like a thick cylinder of craft dough being pressed together on both ends.
- Picture the upper fibers of the psoas gliding down and the lower fibers of the psoas gliding up against slight resistance.

- Visualize the psoas like a sponge filling with water and then being squeezed dry as the psoas condenses.

When using these images, you want to create a subtle shortening along the entire length of the psoas muscle, without moving other parts of the skeleton, such as flexing or side bending the spine, rotating the pelvis, or hiking the hip. As you inhale, imagine filling the whole length of the psoas with your breath. As you exhale, gently activate the psoas by consciously contracting the muscle while visualizing your chosen image. You can move your hands slightly toward each other as a tactile cue that duplicates the shortening and thickening of the muscle. Practice this activation of the psoas for several breaths. You may feel something, just a little, or nothing at all; whatever you are feeling is absolutely perfect. If you can't access a felt experience of the psoas, return to this inquiry another day. Gradually, by repeatedly moving your attention to this deep muscle, you will build a pathway toward a distinct felt experience of it. ::

:: *Psoas Coiling*

Lie on your back in Constructive Rest Position (CRP). Loop a yoga belt around the ball of your right foot and extend the leg toward the ceiling. Keep your left leg bent with the sole of the foot firmly on the floor. On an exhalation, flex the right hip and knee. Use your favorite image from the previous inquiry to visualize the psoas muscle coiling. Feel the upper and lower attachments moving closer together. On your inhalation, imagine that the release of this latent power straightens the leg. Visualize lengthening the psoas as the two ends of the muscle move slightly apart. Repeat these coiling and uncoiling movements several times on the right side. Now straighten both legs along the floor and compare the sensation between your right and left sides. Continue the inquiry on the left side. Finish by relaxing with your legs extended on the floor. Observe the sensations in your body. It is common to experience a sensation of heat in the core of the body after this inquiry.

Once you have learned to engage your psoas lying on your back, experiment with other more challenging positions, such as side lying, all-fours, kneeling, and standing on one or two legs. This work will progressively deepen the repatterning of your movement and will help you to integrate what you have learned into everyday activities, such as walking and running. ⠶

PUTTING IT ALL TOGETHER

In the model that we use in this book, we view the psoas as the primary core muscle that connects all the other core muscles. Without the deeper balance provided by the psoas, premature isolated strength training of the more superficial muscles of the body can be compared to attempting to level a house that has tilted on its foundation by applying plaster to the exterior. The investment you have made in establishing an integrated balance of the psoas has set the stage for you to effectively recruit the secondary core muscles. Working together with the psoas, these secondary core muscles form a cylinder of support throughout the lower and mid-trunk. Over the past two decades, this model of a core cylinder of support has been generated by research into spinal and pelvic stability.[1] The respiratory and pelvic diaphragms form the top and bottom of the cylinder. The front is formed by the deepest

abdominal muscle, the transverse abdominis. The back is supported by one of the strongest spinal muscles, the multifidus. The psoas is the perfect anatomical structure to act as a diagonal strut that connects and reinforces the four quadrants of the cylinder: top to bottom, back to front. This arrangement stabilizes both the lumbar spine and the pelvis (Illustration 24).[2] All of these muscles co-contract in a functioning cylinder of support. When one or more fails to fire in proper sequence, the superficial abdominal muscles are more than happy to take over. The unfortunate result is compromised stability in the lumbar spine and pelvis.

The secondary core muscles work best in concert with a pliant and strong psoas. You can think of your psoas as *the leader of the pack*; when it contracts, it signals the other core muscles to step up to the plate and help with the job. Where are these auxiliary core muscles and what do they do? How do they work together to stabilize the lower back? And what is the function of each member of the cylinder of support? Let's begin by outlining the main players.

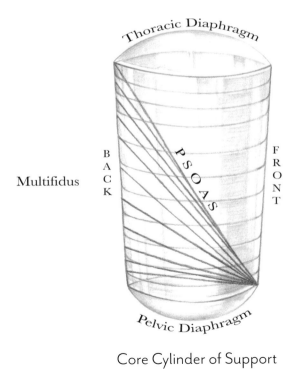

Core Cylinder of Support

ILLUSTRATION 24:
The psoas is the perfect anatomical structure for connecting the four quadrants of the core cylinder of support.

⠿ Tracing the Cylinder of Support

Trace your fingers from your pubic bone up the central line of your abdomen until you reach the sternum (use Illustration 24 as your guide). Imagine a girdle of support with circular fibers that extend from that central line around the entire circumference of the lower trunk. This is the **transverse abdominis** (TA). As you reach the tip of the sternum (xiphoid process), spread your hands to trace around the perimeter of the base of the rib cage, tracing the location of the double-domed **diaphragm**. Move your hands from the front of the rib cage to the back of the body to the level just above the waist on either side of your spine. From this point, sweep your hands all the way down your back to the sacrum, tracing the location of the lumbar **multifidus**. Continue down the sacrum to your tailbone (coccyx), tracing around the pelvic floor or **pelvic diaphragm** (from the coccyx in the back to the pubic bone in the front). To complete the loop, sweep your hands back up the abdomen to your navel. Now slide your hands to the back of the body to the juncture between the thoracic and lumbar spine at the base of the rib cage. It is here that the long tendons of the diaphragm anchor to the lumbar spine and interweave with the origin of **psoas major**. Trace the diagonal bridge from the back of the body down to the front of the pelvis finishing with the fingertips resting on the insides of the thighs where psoas major and the iliacus attach to the lesser trochanter of the femur.

Now let's look at the individual components of the cylinder of support. ⠿

The Thoracic Diaphragm: You already have had an extensive introduction to the anatomy of the thoracic diaphragm in Chapter Two. The most important thing to remember as you learn to build core strength is that the diaphragm co-contracts with the psoas. This is why it's so useful to integrate breathing with the movements in the inquiries and practices that follow.

Transverse Abdominis: The abdominal muscles comprise four layers. Moving from the outer to the inner layer, they are the rectus abdominis, the external obliques, the internal obliques, and the transverse abdominis. Although all of these muscles contribute to core stability, TA is considered to be absolutely crucial to the stabilization of the lumbar spine. Understanding the anatomy of this muscle gives us key insights into how it works to provide this support. In the front of the body, a long fibrous band of tissue called the **linea alba** extends from the xiphoid process (tip of the sternum) all the way down to the pubic symphysis. Note the four points of origin in Illustration 25A. The horizontal fibers of TA extend laterally off the linea alba with fibers attaching to six slips on the inner surface of the cartilage of the 7th to 12th ribs 25A**(1)**. Note that these fibers interweave with the costal part of the thoracic diaphragm. TA also attaches to the inner lip of the iliac crest 25A**(2)**, the anterior superior iliac spine 25A**(3)**, and to the inguinal ligament 25A**(4)** (Illustration 25A). Essentially, TA forms a deep pelvic corset that wraps horizontally all the way from the front of the abdomen to the back of the body (Illustration 25B).

In the back of the body, TA attaches to the transverse processes of the lumbar spine via the medium of the thoracolumbar fascia (Illustration 25C). You'll get an even better understanding of how this works by taking another look at the lumbar spine in cross-section (Illustration 26). You can see not only how the thoracolumbar fascia connects TA to the spine, but also how the fascia envelops the intrinsic muscles of the back. It is this clever arrangement that gives TA such a central role in lumbar stabilization. If you have ever

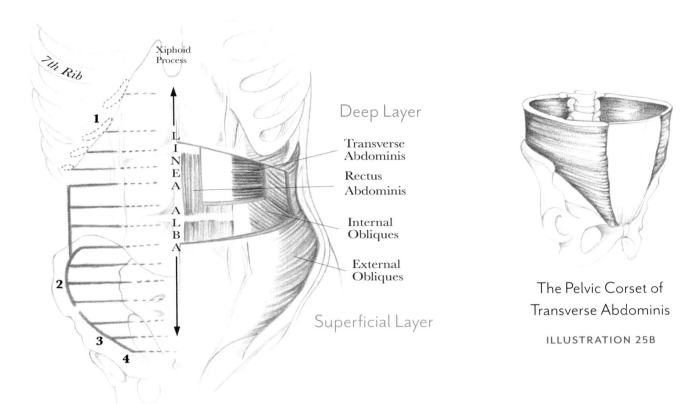

7th Rib

Xiphoid
Process

1

2

3

4

LINEA ALBA

Deep Layer

Transverse
Abdominis

Rectus
Abdominis

Internal
Obliques

External
Obliques

Superficial Layer

Transverse Abdominis
Origins and Insertions

ILLUSTRATION 25A

The Pelvic Corset of
Transverse Abdominis

ILLUSTRATION 25B

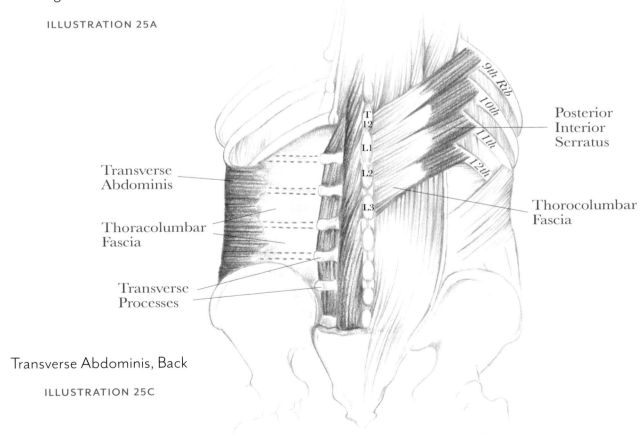

9th Rib

10th

11th

12th

T 12

L1

L2

L3

Posterior
Interior
Serratus

Thorocolumbar
Fascia

Transverse
Abdominis

Thoracolumbar
Fascia

Transverse
Processes

Transverse Abdominis, Back

ILLUSTRATION 25C

Front Body

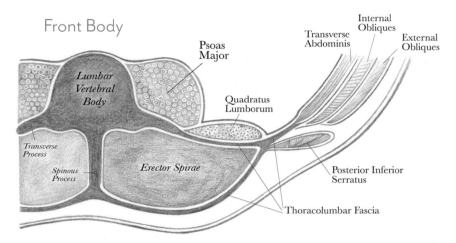

Psoas
Major

Internal
Obliques

Transverse
Abdominis

External
Obliques

Lumbar
Vertebral
Body

Quadratus
Lumborum

Transverse
Process

Spinous
Process

Erector Spirae

Posterior Inferior
Serratus

Thoracolumbar Fascia

Back Body

ILLUSTRATION 26: Psoas Major in Cross-Section

ridden a bicycle down a steep and bumpy slope, you know that as the bicycle picks up speed and begins to totter, you must brace the handlebars to keep the bike steady. If you think of the transverse processes as the little handle bars of the lumbar vertebrae, as TA contracts, the horizontal pull of the thoracolumbar fascia helps to prevent excessive motion in the lumbar vertebrae and stabilizes this vulnerable area of the spine. This is particularly important when lifting weight or when extending the limbs away from the body, such as when you reach to grasp a cup off of a high shelf.

Activating Your Transverse Abdominis

A simple way to feel TA, is to place your hands around the sides of your waist and clear your throat or cough. To train deliberate activation of TA, lie in Constructive Rest Position. Place your fingertips on your abdomen just inside the hip bones. On an exhalation, activate the horizontal fibers of TA between your hands by visualizing the two hip bones moving toward each other as if you are zipping up a pair of tight jeans. Relax your efforts on your inhalation. Repeat several times. You will know whether it is TA activation if you feel a slow swelling up of the muscle underneath your fingers. The common instruction to "move the navel toward the spine" usually results in an activation of the more superficial layers of the abdominal muscles. When you switch on the more superficial abdominal muscles, the sensation will be sharper, quicker, and harder than the sensation of the deeper TA.

Posterior Inferior Serratus—The Secret Helper: Before we leave TA, take a moment to look carefully at the cross-section illustration again (Illustration 26). You'll see that another muscle connects to the spine via the thoracolumbar fascia—the little-known posterior inferior serratus (PIS). This muscle arises from the thoracolumbar fascia in the region of the 12th thoracic vertebrae and the 1st–3rd lumbar vertebrae and extends to the lower ribs, attaching from the 12th to the 9th rib (Illustration 25C). It depresses the lower ribs (particularly on forced exhalation), and indirectly, this action draws the base of the shoulder blades down the back. This anchoring of the rib cage and shoulder blades helps to prevent the upper back from rounding forward. A number of other muscles co-contract with PIS, and their group effort contributes to spinal stabilization. Activating PIS can switch on the latissimus dorsi muscles, which overlay PIS and also connect to the thoracolumbar fascia. Another co-contractor, the lower trapezius muscle, overlaps spinal attachments with PIS from T9 to T12 and is directly involved in moving the shoulder blades down the back. Because PIS connects via the tho-racolumbar fascia to the spine, *when you switch on PIS, it can signal TA to switch on as well.* Engaging PIS and these other muscular "friends" can be essential for activities like horseback riding and martial arts, for which "holding your ground" is imperative to core balance. ⠿

⠿ *Activating Your Posterior Inferior Serratus and Friends*

Stand with your feet slightly wider than your hips, with your knees bent and your arms in front of you as if you're holding a heavy tray. Clench your fists with your thumbs up; then draw your fists slightly upward and your elbows down-ward, making a V shape between the lower and upper arm. On an extended exhalation, con-sciously draw the base of your shoulder blades downward while at the same time anchoring your pelvis toward the ground. Feel how this action lit-erally plugs you into the ground, making it quite difficult for anyone to knock you off balance.

Working with a partner can give you an even better understanding of how powerful engaging these synergistic muscles can be. Return to your power stance with your partner standing directly in front of you. Your partner will take hold of your hands and with gradually increasing pres-sure, try to pull you forward. If you can maintain the strong engagement that keeps the base of the rib cage drawn downward and shoulder blades descending, your partner will find it difficult to pull you forward and knock you off balance. Then allow these muscles to relax, letting the base of your shoulder blades lift upward. Notice how your partner can instantaneously pull you off balance.

Multifidus: You already are familiar with the multifidus muscles, which were introduced in Chapter Two (pages 17–18). The psoas provides deep support to the front of the spine, and the multifidus provide deep support to the back of the spine. This extensive network of muscles relays up the spine from the sacrum to the base of the neck, with its fibers most densely distrib-uted in the lower back (Illustration 27). You can visualize it as the laces of the corset of the TA. When the multifidus contracts, it pulls on the thoraco-lumbar fascia and narrows the waist, like a corset being tightened. Like the psoas muscles,

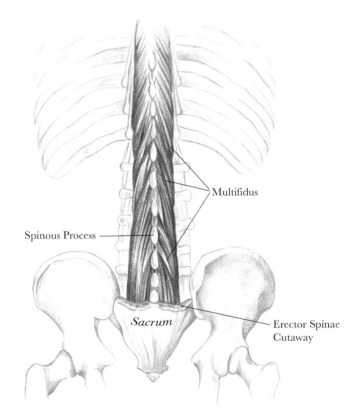

Multifidus

ILLUSTRATION 27

the multifidus is capable of producing extension, lateral flexion, and rotation of the spine, but the primary role of the multifidus is to stabilize and control motion between the vertebral segments. You could think of the multifidus as intricate scaffolding for your spine. This inner support keeps the spine upright and reduces pressure on the intervertebral disks.[3] The multifidus also works in concert with the abdominal muscles by opposing their action of flexion and rotation. Studies have shown that the multifidus muscles are recruited *before* any action such as lifting. This anticipatory contraction stabilizes the spine and protects it from injury. Chronic back pain sufferers consistently show significant reduction of this preemptive engagement.[4]

The multifidus also can assist with the stabilization of the sacroiliac joint. When the multifidus fires, it tends to extend the lumbar spinal muscles and pull the top of the sacrum into a slight anterior tilt. This is called *nutation*. When the muscles of the pelvic floor at the bottom of the cylinder of support engage, they pull the sacrum into a slight posterior tilt. This is called *counternutation*. Both nutation and counternutation are tiny movements of the sacrum within the pelvis and do not move the pelvis itself. Coactivation of both the multifidus and the pelvic floor muscles (i.e., extension and flexion occurring simultaneously) helps to keep the sacrum in a neutral position.

Researcher Richard L. Lieber has shown that the multifidus has a unique molecular structure, which makes these fibers stiffer than any others in the body. Because of this unique design, the multifidus turns out to be the strongest muscle in the back. Most muscles weaken as they are lengthened: when the spine is flexed and the multifidus is elongated, it actually becomes stronger.[5]

Activating Your Multifidus

In a standing position, place the fingertips of both hands on either side of your spine in the deepest part of your lumbar curve. Imagine that you have a heavy dinosaur tail and activate the muscles underneath your fingers as if you are lifting the tail. Activate and release the muscles several times. Alternatively, visualize the laces of a corset being pulled tighter and tighter. You will feel the multifidus contracting beneath your fingers. Practice activating the multifidus in other positions, such as when you are side lying or on all-fours.

The Pelvic Floor: The pelvic floor is a relatively recent evolutionary event. In quadrupeds such as dogs and cats, the floor of the body is the abdominal wall and the front of the thorax; almost no weight rests on the pelvic floor. When we evolved to stand upright, the weight of the abdominal organs shifted to the pelvic floor. The muscles enclosing the lower pelvic inlet now needed to be reinforced and made thicker to contain the organs within the pelvic basin. Remember that the psoas also radically shifted its relationship to gravity in this progression from quadruped to biped.

Although the intricacies of the pelvic floor are outside the scope of this book, it's helpful to find the landmarks of the terrain by locating the tailbone (coccyx) in the back, the pubic bone in the front, and the two sitting bones (ischial tuberosities). These four points form the markers of the pelvic diamond. The pelvic floor has two main layers: a deeper layer is called the **levator ani** and runs from the front to the back and sides of the diamond. The **pubococcygeus** is part of this group of muscles. These muscles are known as the **pelvic diaphragm**, and they form the floor of the core cylinder of support (Illustration 28).

The more superficial layer is called the **urogenital diaphragm** and runs from side to side. Only the deeper layer of the pelvic floor muscles con-

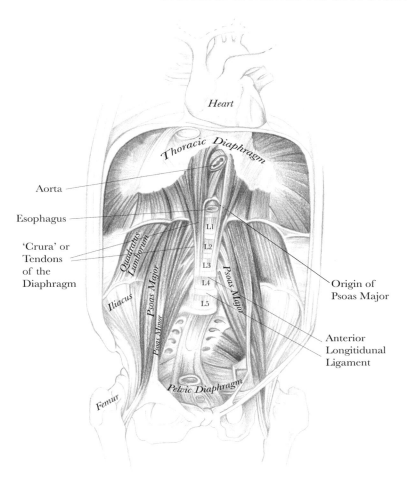

The Pelvic Diaphragm

ILLUSTRATION 28

tributes to core stability. The pelvic diaphragm sits like a muscular sling within the bony inlet at the base of the pelvis. A healthy and well-toned pelvic floor contains the abdominal organs, supports easeful and pleasurable sexual activity, and assists in the movements of defecation.

The pelvic floor is subtly responsive to the movements of the thoracic diaphragm, expanding and softening when the thoracic diaphragm descends on inhalation, and naturally condensing and tonifying when the thoracic diaphragm ascends on exhalation. Thus, the most direct means of learning to engage the pelvic floor muscles is to heighten ones awareness of easeful Diaphragmatic Breathing and to use this awareness while practicing movement and Yoga postures.

For instance, as one lifts the pelvis off of the floor from CRP, exhaling during this lifting phase can elicit a natural tonification of the pelvic floor to support the action.

The natural tonus of the pelvic floor can be compromised by events such as prolonged trauma during childbirth or sustained work involving heavy lifting. Weakness of these muscles can be a causative factor in urinary incontinence in common scenarios such as sneezing, picking up a child, or laughing. Lack of tone in the pelvic floor also can manifest as a collapse of the internal organs such that the cervix may even hang below the opening of the vagina. The common prevailing wisdom is that every pelvic floor problem is caused by looseness or slackness, presumably an inevitable consequence of the aging process. Yet, if the muscles are too tight, difficulties with the pelvic floor can arise in men and in women. Poor posture, as well as sitting and standing that is not self-supported, can be a major contributing factor to a pelvic floor that is too slack or too tight. Certainly, if you experience issues such as daily incontinence or pain during intercourse, we advise seeing a specialist who can accurately assess, diagnose, and advise you on the best course of treatment. We also thoroughly recommend the work of Eric Franklin, author of *Pelvic Power*,[6] and of U.S. Yoga teacher Leslie Howard, who is paving the way toward a more enlightened approach to understanding and healing the pelvic floor.[7] ::

:: Activating Your Pelvic Floor

Sit on a folded blanket so that the pelvis and lumbar spine are in a neutral position, with the weight centered on your sitting bones. You will be sitting on the center of your sitting bones. Bring your attention to the perineum of the pelvic floor (the area between the genitals in the front and the anus in the back). Place a very soft ball, a quarter-inflated Muscle Release (MR Ball),[8] or a folded wash cloth or yoga belt under your perineum. As you inhale, allow the pelvic floor to relax downward into the ball. As you exhale, gently lift the perineum away from the ball, using *only 20 percent* effort. Alternatively, you can activate the pelvic floor by visualizing a broad smile lifting the abdomen just above the pubic bone and spreading to the pelvic bones on either side. It's essential that you do not clench your buttocks, round your back, or tighten and lift your shoulders. When you isolate and engage the pelvic diaphragm, you will feel a deep inner lift that occurs from the front to the back of the body as well as from side to side. Try this exercise for five breaths, relaxing as you inhale and activating the pelvic floor as you exhale.

If you sit for your work, notice whether you round your back when you sit in a chair. This can contribute to prolapse of the organs and inadequate tone in the pelvic floor. Similarly, arching your back and sitting on the edge of your seat can cause the internal organs to fall forward and create too much laxity in the pelvic floor. Notice that when you lean heavily against the back of the chair, all the core muscles tend to switch off. When you sit with your back *resting lightly* against your chair, or completely self-supported, you can strengthen your core just by sitting correctly.

Switching on the Core Cylinder of Support: At some time in your everyday activities, you will have learned that when you pick up a heavy parcel or bag, holding the weight as close as possible to your body, reduces potential stress to your back. When the core of your body is stronger, it is possible to extend weight farther and farther away from your center without strain. A dancer's ability to extend and hold her leg in the air is dependent on having exceptional core strength. Ultimately, the core of the body provides a nexus around which the limbs coordinate their action. In a person with extraordinary core integration, this action happens naturally and without conscious mental effort. To reestablish this natural ease, however, may first require practicing movements slowly and consciously until the engagement of the core once again becomes innate. The following ideokinetic exploration is an excellent way to begin this process. ::

⠿ *The Figure-8 Loop—Engaging the Core through Dynamic Imagery* ⋯⋯⋯⋯⋯⋯⋯⋯⋯

If we asked you to engage your TA, multifidus, pelvic floor, and psoas muscles simultaneously, you would find it hard to translate these instructions into a felt experience. The Figure-8 Loop is a clever dynamic image that bypasses this awkward cognitive process and gives you access to the felt sensation of the core muscles engaging.[9] The primary purpose of the visualization of the loop is to find a neutral pelvic position and to be able to sustain this powerful position as a stable hub from which to extend your limbs. For instance, while on all-fours, you should be able to reach your left arm and right leg off the floor without changing the shape or the position of the lumbar spine and pelvis. The practice of the Figure-8 Loop is especially helpful for hypermobile people who may struggle to find core stability, but the practice should not result in tucking the tailbone under and flattening the lower back.

Stand in bare feet or supportive shoes on a hard floor or firm carpet. Bring your hands to rest on your navel center (Illustration 29A). In your mind's eye, dive through the abdomen, crossing transversely through the body so that you arrive at the top of the sacrum. Bring your hands to rest on your sacrum. Now trace your fingers down the back of the sacrum through to the curved tip of the tail. Continue by tracing from the tail, around the pelvic floor arriving at the pubic bone. Now travel up the abdomen back to the navel as if zipping up a pair of snug jeans. This forms the bottom of the Figure-8 Loop. Run through this imaginary loop several times, feeling the musculature engage down the lumbar spine, up through the pelvic floor, and back to the navel.

Continue your exploration by diving back into the navel center, this time crossing transversely up to the base of the kidneys and lower ribs. Place your hands just above your back waist. Lightly trace up around the back of the body, over the top of the head, and down the face as though you

were putting a hood over your head. Continue down the sternum to the xiphoid process (tip of the breastbone), and complete the loop by connecting back to the navel center. You may want to imagine that you are tying a loose knot between the tip of the sternum and the navel center so that the whole front of the abdominal wall switches on.

Once you have traced the Figure-8 Loop and can feel the activation of your inner core muscles,

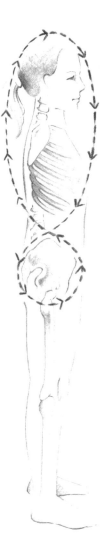

The Figure-8 Loop

ILLUSTRATION 29A

you can extend the loop to connect your body with the earth beneath you and to the space above you (Illustration 29B). Begin the loop as before, but this time as you come down the sacrum and tail, extend the loop down the back of the legs and heels all the way to the ground and to the center of the earth, some 4,000 miles away.[10] Trace this pathway by brushing with your hands all the way to the soles of the feet. Then come back up through the earth, up through the soles of your feet to the inner thighs, and to the front of both legs, arriving back at the pelvic floor and the pubic bone. Continue the loop up the abdomen, diving back into the navel and through to the back of the trunk. As you continue up the back of the body to the top of the head, extend the loop up into the space above you into infinity by reaching the arms upward. Then trace the hands back down your head, face, and sternum, arriving at your navel center.

As you extend the loop to include your relationship with the earth and space, you are learning

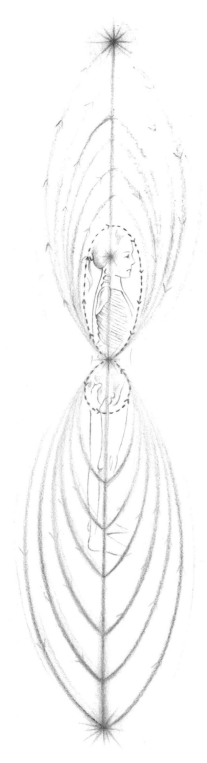

Building the Energetic Core

ILLUSTRATION 29B

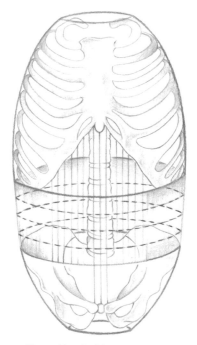

Core Body Engagement
through Rib Cage–Pelvic Balance

ILLUSTRATION 30

how to calibrate your microcosmic human body with the macrocosmic universe around you. This is the beginning of feeling the power of the *hara*, or energetic core, a practice that martial artists, dancers, and other supreme athletes hone over a lifetime. Connecting this energetic center to your environment can radically change your experience of activities, such as walking, running, skiing, and horseback riding, and can give potency to simple practices such as Yoga postures.

The lower part of the Figure-8 Loop provides containment and strength to the pelvic area, whereas the upper part of the loop supports the expression of levity and lightness of the spine into space. Connecting the upper and lower body is crucial for force transmission. When the "up bucket" of the pelvis and the "down bucket" of the rib cage are in a neutral position, these two structures have a functional relationship with one another (Illustration 30). When the tip of the sternum and pubic bone are drawn too far apart, the abdominal wall switches off, causing a telltale paunch. We find that many Yoga students have been taught to "open their chest" by lifting the base of the rib cage, squeezing the shoulder blades together, and drawing the arms behind the natural line of the shoulder girdle. These actions cause a deep hinge in the upper lumbar spine and can switch off the abdominal wall. When the rib cage is balanced over the pelvis, and the distance between the sternum and pubic bone is optimal, the abdominal wall magically switches on. You can achieve this balance by broadening your shoulders (rather than pulling them back), while simultaneously keeping the lower rim of the rib cage contained over the upper rim of the pelvis. Using the Figure-8 Loop image will help you to find this balance.

When you first install the loop, it is useful to continue to use your hands to trace through the pathway, brushing your body lightly to give yourself a somatic imprint of the directions of release and engagement. You can now use this image when fine-tuning your posture or while practicing any Yoga posture or exercise that requires core stability, such as Half Downward Facing Dog (*Ardha Adho Mukha Svanasana*; see page 103).

The Figure-8 Loop Mantra: Use the Figure-8 Loop to establish a neutral pelvic position *before* you begin any exercise or Yoga posture. Then, as you move or change position, notice whether the stability of your core has been affected by the challenge of the movement. You can mindfully integrate this awareness with the cycles of your breath. As you inhale, focus on aligning your head with your tail through the axis of your spine. As you exhale, elongate, open, or deepen into the movement (how you do this will be determined by the specific movement or posture with which you are working). At the end of the exhalation, pause briefly. During this pause, stabilize your body once again, continuing to use the Figure-8 Loop image. If you have discovered another action that works to give you stability, engage that action. Then you can use your breath and the mantra together.

INHALE   Align the head to the tail.

EXHALE   Open, elongate, and deepen (you may want to choose one of these words)

PAUSE   Stabilize (apply the Figure-8 Loop or another stabilizing action)

REPEAT . . .

In this way, you can challenge yourself to maintain your stability even as you are opening your body. In the beginning, you may find that you oscillate between increasing your range of motion followed by loss of stability, followed by finding your center again. Eventually, you will master this process so that you are able to open your body while simultaneously remaining stable.

⠿ *Yield Supports Push Supports Reach*

Stand with your feet slightly wider than your hips. Center the pelvis between the two legs. As you shift your weight onto the right leg, bend the right knee and yield your weight over that foot. Push off from the right foot, shifting the weight to the left leg. Yield your weight over the left foot, while maintaining the neutral position of the pelvis. Imagine the legs and pelvis as the conduit for a bouncing ball that touches the ground with each yield and then bounces off the ground with the push off, traveling up the leg, through the hip socket, through the bridge of the pelvis, and down into the other leg and foot. This is a qualitatively different action than mechanically bending and straightening the knee joints. Repeat several times.

Complete this inquiry by standing with the weight even between the two feet. Now bend both knees as you yield through both feet. Push off to straighten both legs. Imagine the force coming up from the legs, moving into the pelvis, streaming into the psoas muscles, and "launching" the spine into space. You can visualize the push off from the feet like the ground reaction force that lifts a spaceship into takeoff. Keep the pelvis centered as you straighten the legs so that the pelvis can "receive" the force from the legs and transmit it to the spine. You can now use this practice during standing Yoga postures or the practice of Sun Salutations (*Suryanamaskar*). ⠿

❖ *Using Sound and Breathing to Increase Core Awareness*

Author and riding instructor Mary Wanless suggests these exercises for increasing your awareness of your core abdominal muscles.[11] Begin by lying comfortably in CRP. Place your hands gently on your lower abdomen and clear your throat (or cough). As you do so, you will feel a more specific sense of the engagement of your abdominal muscles.

Lower Abdomen: Place your hands on your lower abdomen. As you exhale make the sound *psst, psst.* Feel the activity of the abdominal muscles below the navel. Repeat several times.

Mid-Abdomen: Now bring your hands to the area around your navel. Make the sound *sssh,*

sssh. This will help you feel the middle abdominal area. Repeat several times.

Upper Abdomen: Now place your hands on your upper abdomen beneath your rib cage. As you exhale make the sound *grr, grr.* This will help you feel the upper abdominal area as well as the sides and back of the waist. This sound may also make your feel powerful!

As you move through the sequences that follow, experiment with using these sounds on your exhalation as a way to refine your awareness of where and what you are engaging. You also can return to the *WHO* breath at any time when you wish to feel stronger core engagement (see page 45). ❖

PRACTICES

Core Toning with Block

Benefits

- Strengthens transverse abdominis.
- Assists in closure of the sacroiliac joint by strengthening the adductors.
- Heightens awareness of the pelvic floor.

Contraindications

- None.

You'll Need

- A yoga mat covered with a folded blanket.
- A yoga belt.
- A yoga block or thick book.

Why: The focal point of this exercise is integrating your breathing with the engagement of TA.

How: Lie in CRP. Place a yoga block (at its narrowest width) between your knees. Place the pads of the fingers on your lower abdomen just inside the hip bones. Inhale and as you exhale sequentially press the feet into the ground and gently hold (but do not grip) the block between the knees to activate the adductors muscles of the inner thighs. Imagine your torso as a cylinder; narrow the middle of the cylinder as you exhale (Figure 28). You may wish to add the *WHO* sound as you exhale to accentuate the activation of transverse abdominis. Keep your feet and back on the floor and keep the lumbar spine in neutral. The lumbar curve may flatten *slightly* as it elongates, but your aim is not to press your lumbar spine onto the floor. On an inhalation, sequentially relax the abdomen, pelvic floor, inner thighs, and feet without dropping the block. Repeat eight times.

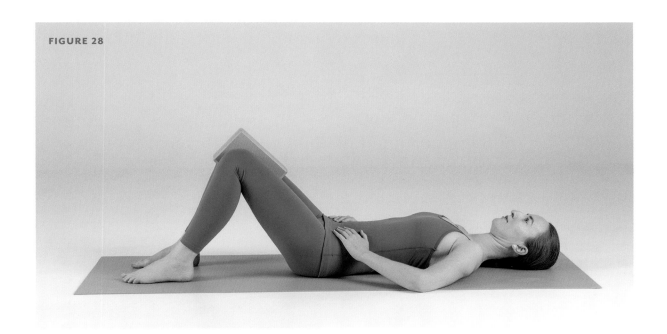

FIGURE 28

Reclining Bound Angle (*Supta Baddha Konasana*)

Benefits

- Improves awareness of the pelvic floor muscles by both relaxing and tonifying the pelvic diaphragm.
- Tonifies the vagina and clarifies the action of Kegel exercises.
- Improves blood flow to the organs of the lower abdomen.

Contraindications

- Do not practice if you are bleeding heavily during menstruation.

You'll Need

- A yoga mat cushioned with a blanket.

Why: Many women are given Kegel exercises without any guidance as to *how* to distinguish the muscles of the pelvic floor from the gluteal muscles. This often results in women simply tightening their butt or inner thighs without targeting the muscles of the pelvic floor.

How: Begin in CRP. As you inhale, relax the pelvic floor, abdomen, and inner thighs, and with control, open your knees out to the sides, rocking onto the outer edges of your feet with the soles facing each other (Figure 29). Exhale and bring your knees up to the starting position while consciously tonifying the pelvic floor as you did in the inquiry on pages 112–114.

Try practicing this exercise with one lubricated finger gently inserted into your vagina so that you can feel how these muscles relax and engage as the legs open and close. You'll be amazed how clearly you can feel the vaginal wall engaging by adding the *WHO* sound through gently pursed lips on each exhalation.

At the end of the exhalation, briefly accentuate the muscular contraction. Repeat eight times.

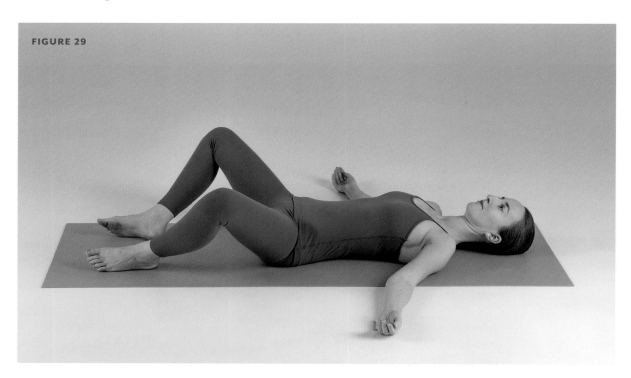

FIGURE 29

The Drawbridge

Benefits

- Enhances core strengthening.
- Specifically activates the deep psoas and decreases habitual overuse of the superficial muscles.
- Is accessible to even those with weak core muscles.

Contraindications

- People with compromised disk health or disk herniation should be cautious.
- Do not practice if you have advanced spondylolisthesis or spinal stenosis, hernia, or acid reflux.

You'll Need

- A yoga mat and blanket.
- A yoga belt.

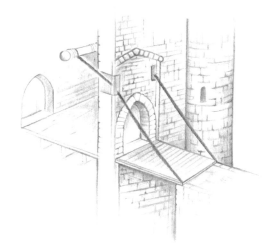

The Drawbridge

ILLUSTRATION 31

Why: Reliance on the *superficial duplicators* during hip flexion is usually an unconscious action. It is only when we become conscious of our habits that we can change them. When you focus your attention precisely on the psoas and its attachments, and use imagery to deliberately initiate the movement, the likelihood is greater that the deeper core muscle will be activated. In the following inquiries, the image of a drawbridge can be used in both eccentric and concentric contractions to bring more precision and refinement to movements of the hip (Illustration 31). These variations of the Drawbridge are progressively more challenging. Start with the first variation and work up to the one that challenges you but does not cause you strain. The first inquiry can help you learn how to relax the superficial duplicators.

How

Variation A with a Belt: Lie on your back with the sacrum centered on a folded blanket. Bend both knees and place the feet flat on the floor. Loop a yoga belt around the shin of the right leg just below the knee. Hold one end of the yoga belt loosely in each hand. Keeping your legs passive like a puppet, use your arm strength to draw the thigh toward the belly so that the right foot lifts a few inches off the floor (Figure 30). Imagine the belt as the chains raising the "drawbridge" of the thigh. Then slowly lower the foot back down to the floor, visualizing the drawbridge being lowered by the chains. Alternate between the passive concentric movement (muscle shortens and contracts) and eccentric movement (muscle lengthens and contracts). It can be a challenge to allow the leg to be moved passively. Monitor and inhibit any habitual impulse to "help" the passive movement: relax the abdominal and quadriceps muscles. Repeat on the other leg. Stay with this variation until all the hip flexors remain relaxed throughout the movement.

Variation B with Knees Drawn: Lie on your back with the pelvis elevated on a folded blanket. Draw both knees into the chest so the pelvis is slightly tucked under. Place your hands at either end of the right psoas muscle. To a count of four, slowly lower the right foot until it touches the floor (Figure 31). Visualize the psoas as chains reeling out and slowly lowering the heavy drawbridge of the thigh. You may find it helpful to use your hands to draw the two points of the attachments apart. Then visualize the chains reeling in and raising the drawbridge of the thigh as you lift the foot and drawn the knee back into the chest. Again, you may find it helpful to use your hands to draw the two points of attachment together. Repeat several times. Then repeat on the other leg. Notice any differences between the two sides. The raising and lowering movements may be coordinated with the phases of the breath.

If you focus on the drawbridge image, eventually any unconscious habit of activating the superficial duplicators will be inhibited and you will learn to initiate flexion and eccentric extension of the hip bones by consciously activating the psoas muscles.

Variation C with Leg Extension: Begin in the same starting position as Variation B with your pelvis on a folded blanket or low bolster with both knees drawn into the chest. Your hands may be placed on the upper and lower abdomen. On an inhalation, extend the right leg up toward the

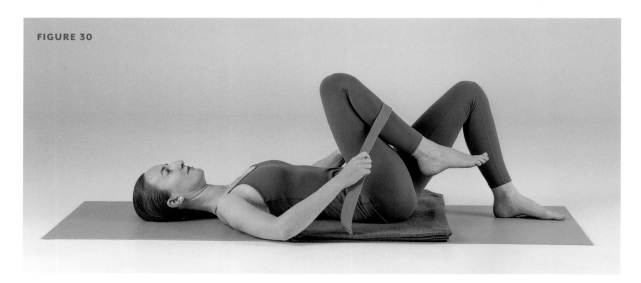

FIGURE 30

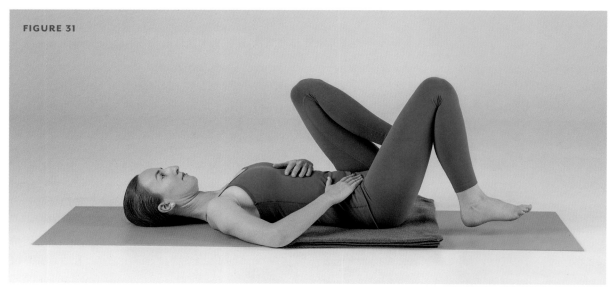

FIGURE 31

ceiling (Figure 32A). On an exhalation, reach out through your heel and slowly lower the leg until it rests briefly on the floor. This movement also can be done incrementally taking several breaths to reach the floor (Figure 32B). As you lower the leg, visualize the lengthening contraction of the psoas between its upper and lower attachments. Use the image of the drawbridge to help you. On your inhalation, bend your right knee, bring it back toward the abdomen and extend the leg toward the ceiling once again. Repeat three to five times. Then repeat on the other leg. Throughout the exercise maintain a neutral lumbar curvature. If your lumbar spine begins to arch away from the floor, this is an indication that your core muscles are not yet strong enough to support the weight of your leg so far from your center. You may need to return to Variation B.

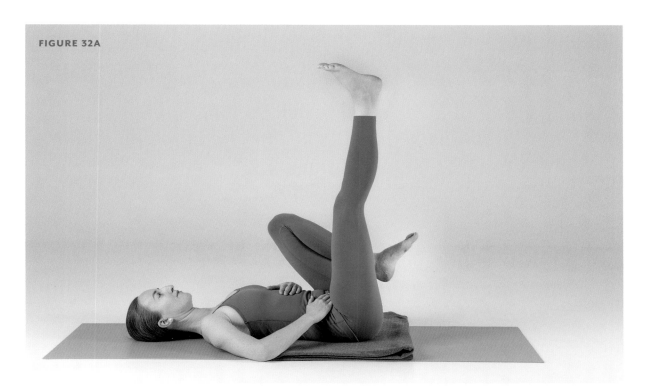

FIGURE 32A

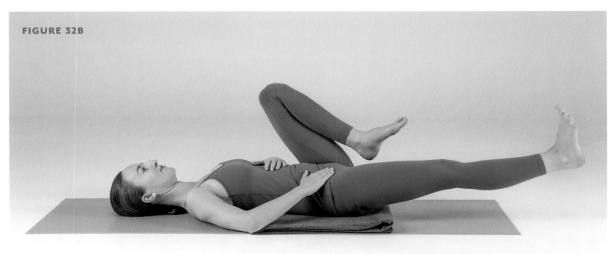

FIGURE 32B

Heel and Toe Touches

Benefits

- Encourages core strengthening, in particular for those with spinal problems.
- Reduces strain on the neck and lower back compared with traditional "crunches" or some Pilates exercises.
- Is accessible to even those with weak core muscles.

Contraindications

- Same as the Drawbridge (see page 121).

You'll Need

- A yoga mat and blanket.

Why: Many approaches to core strengthening place undue strain on the neck and lower back by placing these structures in deep flexion. This deep flexion puts enormous strain on the intervertebral disks and can cause bulging of the annulus (the outer layer of the disk) or even complete rupture of the disk. Ironically, those with compromised spinal health are often the most in need of gaining greater core strength. These exercises, adapted

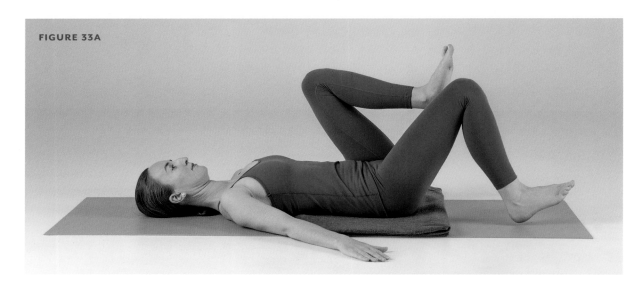

FIGURE 33A

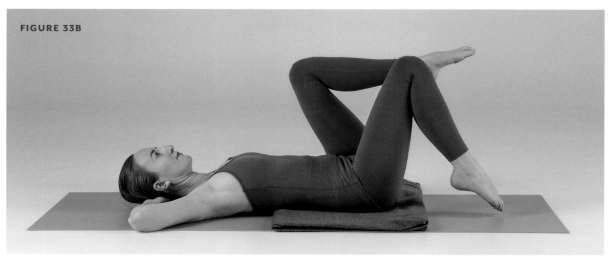

FIGURE 33B

from the work of Sarah Keys, are a safe method for most people.[12] If this practice causes you any discomfort in your back, stop and seek the help of someone competent in spinal rehabilitation.

How

Heel Touches: Place a blanket on top of your yoga mat so that your trunk is cushioned and your feet are placed securely on your yoga mat. Lie down in CRP with your arms on either side of your hips. Alternatively, if you are confident that you already have sufficient core strength, interlace your fingers behind your head. If having the hands behind the head causes you to arch your lower back, or this feels too strenuous on your abdominal muscles, bring your arms back down by your sides. Bring your left knee in toward your chest, and as you start to return your left leg to the floor, simultaneously draw the right leg toward the chest so that the legs pass one another in mid-

air. The heel of your returning foot should *lightly touch* the floor, close to your buttocks, before returning to the knee-to-chest position (Figure 33A). Do not let either foot rest on the floor between excursions, and do not straighten either knee during the exercise. Continue for 60 seconds, moving the legs slowly and with control. Use the image of the drawbridge if you found it helpful.

Toe Touches: You can adapt this exercise so that the toe rather than the heel is touching (Figure 33B). As you get stronger, you can vary the movement by touching the toe to the floor slightly away from the buttocks. Ensure that you are not arching your lower back and that your buttocks are weighted on the floor as you touch the toe to the floor, alternating between the two legs for 60 seconds. When you have completed both rounds, extend both legs along the floor and give the legs a little shake to release the hips and back.

Bridge Pose (*Setu Bandhasana*)

Benefits
- Strengthens the legs and abdominal muscles.
- Releases and strengthens the iliopsoas muscles.
- Strengthens the hamstrings to stabilize the pelvis.

Contraindications
- Not suitable during menstruation because of the inversion of the pelvis.

You'll Need
- A yoga mat and blanket.
- A yoga block.
- An MR Ball.

Why: Lifting the pelvis *slightly* off the floor takes far more control than lifting the whole trunk. Isolating this movement will help you gain control of your pelvis and gradually strengthen the core

muscles. Learning to sequence the action from the ground up—feet, inner thighs, pelvic floor, and abdomen—entrains an awareness of the involvement of the whole body in core engagement. The practice of Bridge Pose also strengthens weak and overstretched hamstring muscles. The hamstrings attach to the sitting bones; contracting them draws the base of the pelvis toward the heels and reduces excessive lumbar curvature.

How

Variation A—Low Bridge Pose: Lie in CRP, and then move the feet closer to your buttocks so that you can use the legs to support the lift of your pelvis off the floor. Place a block or pillow between your knees. Hold the prop lightly with as little effort as possible. As you exhale, press your feet downward, ensuring that the inner edges of your feet are actively in contact with the ground. Pressing the base of the big toe will give you a direct connection to the central axis. This emphasis on keeping the weight on the inner edges of the feet will help you to activate the inner thighs and to engage the muscles of the pelvic floor. Now draw the tailbone toward the pubis, and then lift the pelvis slightly off the floor. Draw the pubic bone toward the navel and check that your navel is *lower* than your pubic bone throughout the exercise (Figure 34A). Keep the upper back and ribs on the floor so that you anchor the base of the rib cage near T12. Inhale, and hold the bridge position. Exhale, and slowly lower your buttocks back to the starting position while reaching the tailbone toward the feet and drawing the abdomen

firmly inward. You may wish to make the *WHO* or *sssh* sounds as you exhale to increase your awareness of the middle of the abdomen. As the pelvis touches the floor, take a full inhalation and completely relax the abdominal wall. Feel how the lumbar spine indents away from the floor. Do not inhibit this natural release of the abdomen and spine. Repeat eight times.

Variation B—Dynamic Bridge Pose: Lie in CRP. To encourage a trampoline-like action, place a half-deflated MR Ball under your pelvis during this exercise (Figure 34B). In this Dynamic Bridge Pose, you will lift your pelvis and spine off the floor as one cohesive unit. Your weight will rest on your shoulders, but be sure to keep the pubic

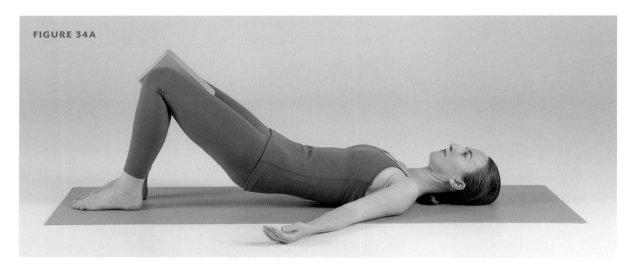

FIGURE 34A

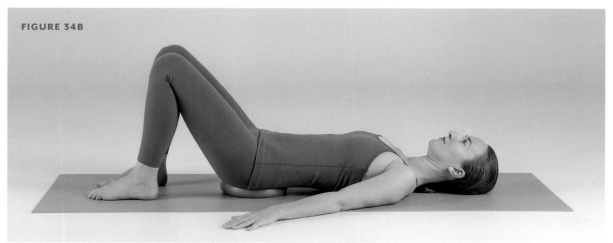

FIGURE 34B

bone higher than your navel. As you inhale, visualize the powerful coiling action of the psoas, and as you exhale, unleash this power and move dynamically up into the Bridge (Figure 34C). On an inhalation lower your pelvis back down to the MR Ball. Repeat several times.

Variation C—High Bridge Pose: Lie in CRP and then adjust your feet so they are close to your buttocks. Place a block or pillow between your knees, using as little effort as possible to hold it. If you require further stabilization, you can experiment with using the cross-belt or the shin-to-thigh technique (page 49–51). This technique is especially useful if you have difficulty keeping your thighs parallel.

On an exhalation, sequentially press the feet and engage the inner thighs and pelvic floor. Reach the tailbone toward the backs of the knees and lift the pelvis, curling the pubic bone toward the navel. Continue to lift the lower back, mid-back, and upper back off the floor until you are resting on your shoulders. Keep the navel slightly *lower* than your pubic bone (Figure 34D). Inhale and hold the Bridge. After five to seven exhalations, incrementally lower the spine toward the floor, pausing and holding the position on your inhalation and moving on your exhalation until the spine is once again resting on the floor. Completely relax all effort for several breaths and then repeat the sequence three times.

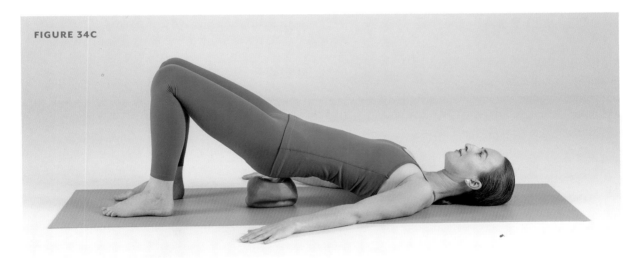

FIGURE 34C

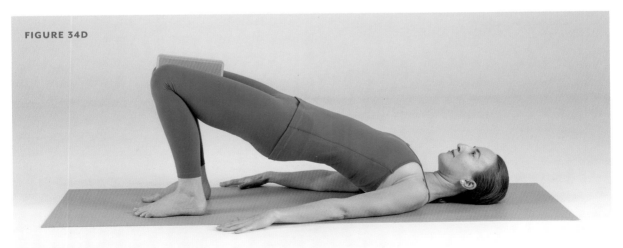

FIGURE 34D

Drawing Circles

Benefits

- Enables you to feel and strengthen transverse abdominis.
- Strengthens weak adductors.
- Is generally safe for those with back problems because it does not place the lower back in flexion.

Contraindications

- None.

You'll Need

- A yoga mat and blanket.

Why: This is a gentle, safe, and effective way to strengthen your abdominal muscles.

How: Lie in CRP. Bring both knees toward the chest, and then open the thighs and lower legs 30 degrees to each side, like opening the two pages of a book. Form a right angle between your thigh and lower leg and point the toes of both feet. Imagine that the whole of each lower leg is a cal-ligraphy pen and that you have a canvas in front of you. Maintaining the position of your thighs, slowly and with control draw two *inwardly* spiraling circles with your lower legs, keeping your toes pointed (Figure 35). Place your fingers just inside your hip bones on your lower abdomen and you will feel the strong activation of the TA muscles, like a deep supportive band across your belly. Experiment with making the circles bigger and smaller. Opening the angle of your thighs to 45 degrees will make the exercise even more challenging. Practice for 60 seconds and then return to CRP. You may wish to do several sets, finishing by extending both legs out along the floor and giving them a little shake.

TIME TO RELAX

It's just as important to learn to relax your core muscles as it is to engage and strengthen them. Use this simple inversion to complete the series.

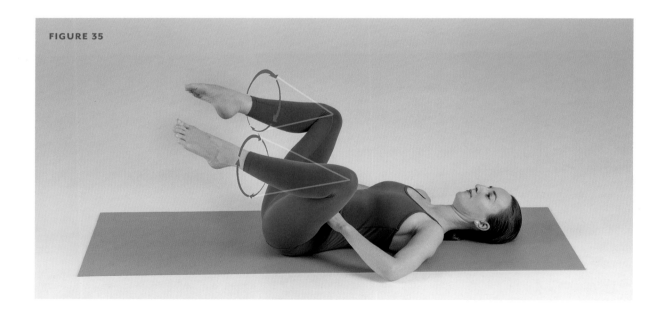

FIGURE 35

The Great Rejuvenator (*Viparita Karani*)

Benefits

- Relaxes the pelvic floor and abdominal muscles.
- Facilitates full Diaphragmatic Breathing.
- Encourages lymphatic drainage to counter water retention in the feet and lower legs.
- Feels deeply relaxing and sedating.

Contraindications

- Avoid if you have high blood pressure, glaucoma, or detached retina.
- Do not practice if you are menstruating.

You'll Need

- A yoga mat.
- A stable chair.
- A bolster or several blankets.
- A yoga belt.

Why: This posture relaxes the abdomen and pelvic floor and places the chest slightly lower than the abdominal organs so that minimal pressure is placed on the diaphragm. The inverted position of the diaphragm tends to favor the ascent of these muscles, supporting the restoration of a full and fluid exhalation. Thus, we return full circle to the importance of Diaphragmatic Breathing in the cylinder of support.

How: Place a chair on your yoga mat, cushioning the seat of the chair with a blanket if necessary. Position a bolster in front of the chair. Sitting on the bolster while facing the chair, tie the upper third of your thighs together with a yoga belt. Lie back with your buttocks on the bolster, your lower legs on the chair, and your neck, head, and shoulders resting on the floor (Figure 36A). If your back is uncomfortable, consider using two folded blankets under the neck, head, and shoulders to reduce the angle of the lower back (Figure 36B).

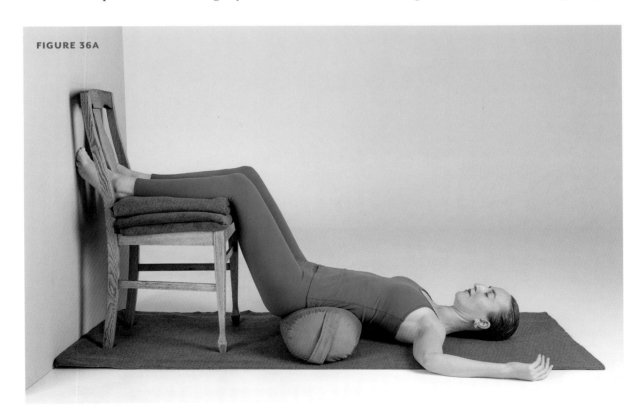

FIGURE 36A

Alternatively, you can lower the height of the pelvis by placing one or two folded blankets under the buttocks instead of a bolster. Completely relax your pelvic floor and abdominal muscles. Observe the interplay of the movement of the breath between your thoracic diaphragm and your pelvic diaphragm. As you inhale, the thoracic diaphragm descends and the pelvic diaphragm relaxes downward. As you exhale, the thoracic diaphragm ascends and the pelvic diaphragm naturally draws upward without any effort on your part. Stay for 7–15 minutes. When you are ready to come out of the pose, slowly push yourself backward off the bolster and rest for several minutes with your knees supported on the bolster and your trunk resting flat on the floor.

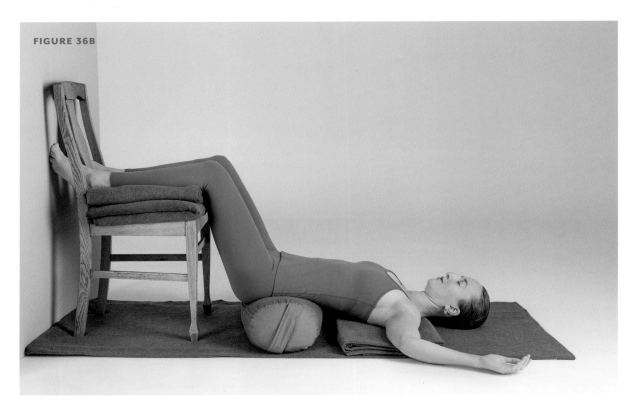

FIGURE 36B

Practice Summary

You can use the practices in this chapter individually or as a practice sequence. If you have a tendency toward hypermobility, consider finishing your exercise routine or Yoga practice with one or two stabilizing exercises each day.

- Core Toning with Block
- Reclining Bound Angle

- The Drawbridge Variations A, B, and C
- Heel and Toe Touches
- Low Bridge Pose Variation A
- Dynamic Bridge Pose Variation B
- High Bridge Pose Variation C
- Drawing Circles
- The Great Rejuvenator

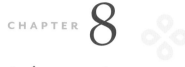

CHAPTER 8

Containment:
How to Safely Open Your Hips

STABILITY AND MOBILITY

ESTABLISHING AND MAINTAINING core stability is especially important if you do practices such as Yoga or dance that require extraordinary mobility of the hips. Keep in mind that the Celestial Design Committee designed the hip socket to be one of the most stable joints in the body. The ability to walk and run long distances without injuring the hips was essential to the survival of Paleolithic man. The depth of the hip socket (acetabulum) and the tremendously strong muscles and ligaments that surround the joint ensure that the femur remains intact and reduces the chance that the hip will dislocate. By comparison, the shoulder joint is a shallow socket with a much greater range of motion that allows for extensive mobility in the arms. This impressive mobility comes at a price—dislocation of this joint is relatively common compared with the hip joint. The inherent stability of the hip means that it is not designed to move beyond certain ranges of motion. If you want to have healthy hips (and knees) later on in life, we strongly advise against trying to move your hips as if they were shoulders in Yoga postures that, for instance, take the feet behind the head. Not only do such movements have the potential to damage the hip itself, the stability of the pelvis and sacroiliac joints suffer the consequences of these extreme movements. We are seeing an alarming trend toward long-time Yoga practitioners and dancers requiring hip replacements at relatively young ages.

CREATING HEALTHY HIP MOBILITY

Reclining Big Toe Pose (*Supta Padangusthasana*) is one of the most common Yoga postures used to release and lengthen the hamstring muscles and to open the hip joints. Variations of this movement are seen in many fitness regimens. When the leg is drawn toward the chest (flexion), opened out to the side (externally rotated), and crossed over the midline (internally rotated), one has an almost complete movement sequence to reestablish full mobility of the hips. These movements are a fantastic investment in keeping your hip joints healthy and mobile, and freely swinging hips indirectly contribute to spinal health.

Because the hamstrings attach to the base of the pelvis, short and tight hamstrings tend to pull the pelvis and lumbar spine into flexion. When this happens, pure iliofemoral movement (i.e., the isolated swing of the femur within the hip socket) is lost, such that every movement of the legs indirectly tugs on the spine. Also, the neutral position of the pelvis becomes distorted, and the psoas and other core muscles are unable to function optimally. We have seen hundreds of Yoga students with back pain experience significant reduction or complete amelioration of their symptoms just by reestablishing hip mobility. That's the good news.

The bad news is that hip-opening movements practiced without stability within the pelvis can destabilize and damage the sacroiliac joint. Recall that the sacroiliac joint has a veritable Fort Knox of ligamentous tissue ensuring that the sacrum and adjoining ilia stay snugly joined. At the same time, the hip joint is the deepest, most stable ball-and-socket joint in the body. When the hip joint is restricted, it can be tempting to try to force the joint open by using the weight of the leg. Frequently, we see students who have had teachers apply external pressure in the form of adjustments to push the hip beyond its natural flexibility. If upon reaching the end of your natural range of motion (something that is determined as much by your bony structure as muscle tightness), you forcefully lever into the joint with the weight of your femur, the femur likely will pry the ilium away from the sacrum. These kinds of actions overstretch the ligaments within the hip socket, can create tearing of the labrum (a thick cartilaginous band of tissue around the perimeter

of the acetabulum that increases hip stability), and can damage the ligaments that hold the sacroiliac joint together. The increased movement you perceive—for instance, getting your knees to the floor in Bound Angle Pose (*Baddha Konasana*)—may be a result of the separation between the ilia and sacrum rather than the opening in the hip socket. This can lead to chronic pelvic instability.

We believe that the forceful opening of the hip bones beyond a healthy range of movement is a strong contributing factor to the epidemic of sacroiliac problems and the rising incidence of labral tears in Yoga practitioners. Once the ligaments in your sacroiliac joint are overstretched, they are overstretched forever. If you suffer from sacroiliac instability, you will need to reinforce the sacroiliac joint through regional muscular support (i.e., you will need much greater core stability to reduce excessive movement within your sacroiliac joint).

Therefore, most of the variations in this chapter place a strong emphasis on keeping the pelvis stable with both buttocks equally weighted on the floor. Your navel remains centered without turning toward the opening leg. Throughout these sequences, it is helpful to consider whether you would be able to let go of the leg that you are stretching without the pelvis rocking to one side. It also may be useful to imagine that you are practicing the sequence in an upright position. A ballet dancer standing at the barre needs to engage the core muscles of her body to control the lift and position of her leg to the front and to the side. When you lie on the floor, the tendency is to disengage core support and to allow your limbs to "flop." If you did this same action while standing, your pelvis would have to turn or you would fall over. By stabilizing the pelvis, you will discover how to differentiate movement at the level of your femur and hip socket rather than opening the hip by prying apart the sacroiliac joint.

INQUIRY: *The Pelvic Reset: Aligning and Stabilizing Your Pelvis*

Before doing a hip-opening practice, it can be helpful to have a kinesthetic sense of optimal alignment and stability in the pelvis and hip sockets. The Pelvic Reset is a self-help osteopathic technique that can realign and stabilize the pelvis so that the heads of the femurs are centered in their sockets. It is sometimes called "The Shotgun" because it can alleviate pelvic, low back, and hip pain generated by a variety of different causes.

Benefits

- Realigns and stabilizes the pelvis.
- Facilitates resolution of sacroiliac joint and low back pain.
- Rebalances hypermobile sacroiliac joints.

Contraindications

- If you have sacroiliac joint pain or instability, you may want to practice this technique only with the legs hip-width apart. To find this neutral alignment, place your two fists side by side between your bent knees and then align your feet and knees. Practicing with the legs wider or narrower than this neutral position may aggravate your sacroiliac joint pain.
- If you experience any discomfort doing this sequence, even with the legs hip-width apart, discontinue the practice and consult your health professional.

You'll Need

- A yoga mat and yoga belt.
- A hard foam yoga block (8 × 15 × 23 cm/3 × 6 × 9 inches); if you don't have a block, improvise with lightweight objects of this approximate size.

Why: If you practice mobilizing, flexibility, or strengthening techniques when your pelvis is misaligned, you may be reinforcing the misalignment. When you do a preliminary practice to realign your pelvis closer to its anatomically correct position, you can achieve the full benefit from the rest of your practice. The Pelvic Reset uses the technique of rhythmical isometric muscle contraction to reposition the pelvic bones. This technique can both decompress a compressed sacroiliac joint and awaken the ligamentous *memory* of joint snugness in a hypermobile sacroiliac joint. If your pelvis tends toward instability, the Pelvic Reset can be used to reestablish pelvic stability after a practice such as hip opening.

How: Start in CRP with the knees and inner feet touching at the midline. For each of the three parts of the Pelvic Reset, keep the following practice notes in mind:

- Synchronize your breath and movement. **Inhale** while you **apply pressure** against the belt or the block and **exhale** as you **release the pressure**.
- Increase or decrease the pressure on the belt or block, in a gradual, smooth, and slow manner.
- Start with a pressure of zero and build to 20 percent effort. Less is more!
- Initiate the movement from your core.
- Before you press outward (abduction), press the inner edge of the foot firmly into the ground. Before you press inward (adduction), press the outer edge of the foot firmly into the ground. This counterbalances the outward or inward movement of the knee and activates the core muscles.

Abduction (Pressing Outward): Follow the next three steps to practice abduction:

A. Fasten your yoga belt halfway between your knees and groin so your inner knees touch. Tighten the belt so it holds your knees together firmly but comfortably (Figure 37A). On an inhalation, press the inner edges of the feet into the floor, and then gently press **out** against the belt. Gradually build up your pressure from zero to 20 percent contraction. As you exhale, gradually release the pressure on the belt. Repeat this pressure-and-release cycle two more times.

B. Loosen the belt so you can move your legs apart, aligning your feet and knees to the width of your hip sockets. For most people, the feet and knees will be approximately 13–18 centimeters (5–7 inches) apart (Figure 37B). Repeat the pressure-and-release cycle three more times, as in A.

C. Loosen the belt so you can move your knees slightly wider than your hips. Move the feet to match the alignment of the knees (Figure 37C). Repeat the pressure-and-release cycle three times.

Adduction (Pressing Inward): Follow the next three steps to practice adduction:

A. Place the widest edge of the foam block between your knees (Figure 37D). On an inhalation, anchor the outer edge of the foot onto the floor and gently press inward against the block, building up to 20 percent effort. Then, gradually release on an exhalation. Practice this cycle three times.

B. Reposition the block with its middle edge between your knees and adjust your feet to align with the knees (Figure 37E). Repeat three times, as in A.

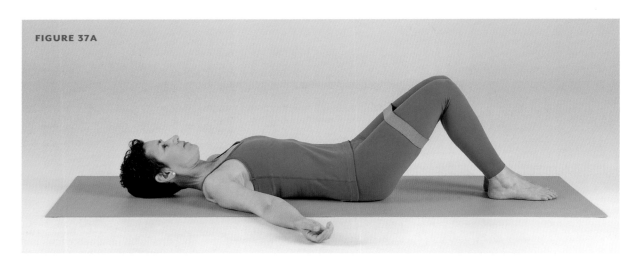

FIGURE 37A

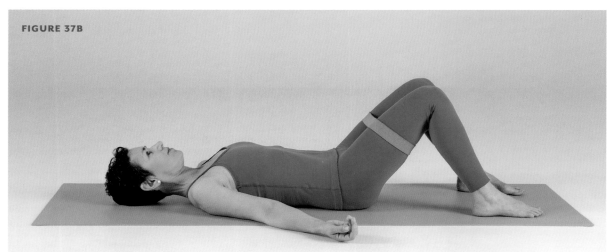

FIGURE 37B

FIGURE 37C

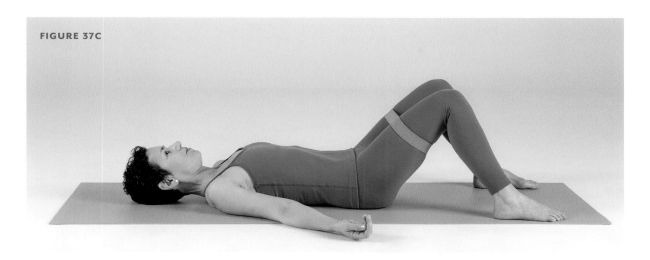

FIGURE 37D

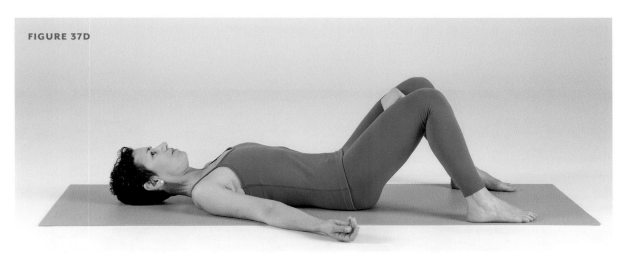

FIGURE 37E

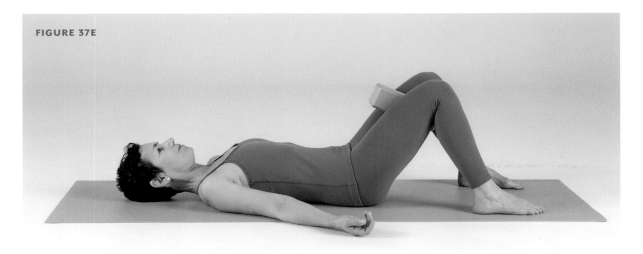

C. Reposition the block with its narrowest edge between your knees and adjust your feet to align with the knees (Figure 37F). Repeat three times.

D. Remove the block and move your feet so the inner edges are touching. Gently press your knees together and release. Repeat three times.

Alternating Abduction and Adduction: To finish the sequence now place either the narrow or middle edge of the block between your knees, whichever feels most comfortable. Tighten the belt so it holds the knees firmly against the block. The block can rest on the belt (Figure 37G). On an inhalation, anchor the outer edge of the foot and gently press **into** the block; then exhale and gently release the pressure. On the next inhalation, anchor the inner edge of the foot and gently press **out** into the belt. As you exhale release the pressure. Now alternate, pressing inward and then outward three times. Always end with an extra movement pressing **into** the block.

Finish the Sequence: Practice Dynamic Bridge Pose (*Setu Bandhasana*) four or five times (Figure 38). The belt and block will help you maintain good alignment between the pelvis and legs. You also can use the cross-belt technique (see pages 49–51) to stabilize both the pelvis and legs. After practicing Bridge Pose, remove the belt and block

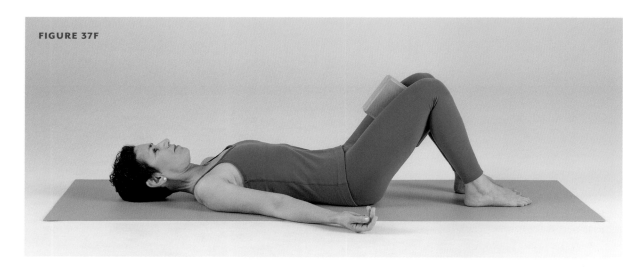
FIGURE 37F

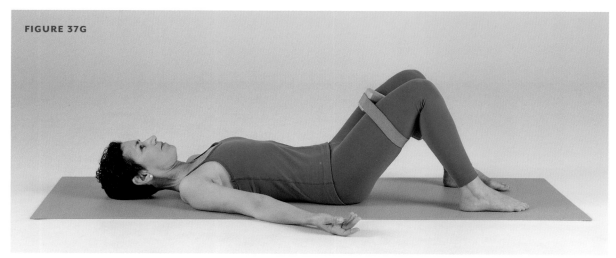
FIGURE 37G

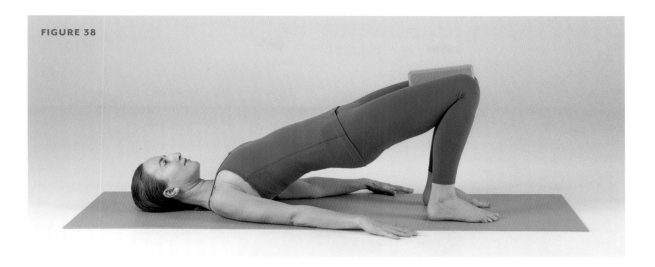

FIGURE 38

and lie on your back for a few moments to notice any interesting effects from this practice. Now stand up and stroll around the room. Do you feel greater comfort in your sacroiliac joint and lower back? Do you notice any changes to your physical balance or your ease in walking? What else do you notice? ⁝

PRACTICES

Mobilizing the Hips: Supine Big Toe Pose (*Supta Padangusthasana*)

Benefits
- Improves hip mobility and lengthens the hamstrings.
- Indirectly improves spinal health by removing the "pull" on the spine from rusty hip joints.
- May bring the pelvis back to a centered position to support good posture and ease in walking.

Contraindications
- People with hip prosthesis should consult their health professional before practicing hip-mobilizing exercises.

You'll Need
- A yoga mat and blanket.
- A yoga belt.

Why: This is one of the easiest and most beneficial movement sequences you can do throughout your life to maintain healthy hips, good posture, and a happy spine. Because the movement is practiced supine, it takes little energy and can be a relaxing way to start or finish your day.

How

Variation A with Hip Flexion: Lie in CRP. On an exhalation, bend your right knee and bring your right leg toward your chest. Hold the back of the thigh or bring your hands around your shin. Take several breaths, allowing the leg to make small excursions away from the chest (on the inhalation) and toward the chest (on the exhalation). Once you have synchronized your movement with your breath, slowly straighten the right leg placing the belt around the *ball* of the foot (Figure 39A). If your thigh is not at 90 degrees or more, bend the thigh just enough to bring the leg beyond

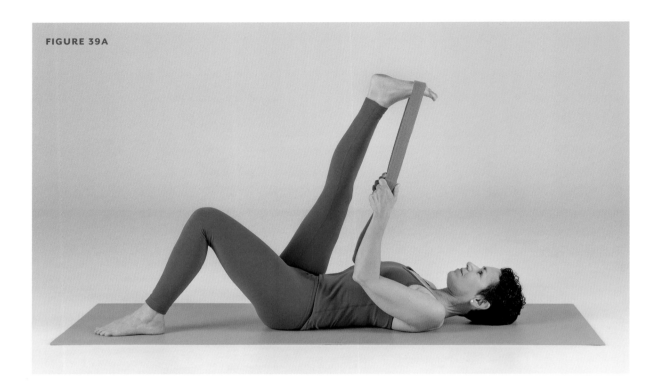

FIGURE 39A

perpendicular to the floor. Keep your thigh at this angle as you *attempt* to straighten the leg. You will feel a strong sensation down the back of the leg whether or not you straighten the leg completely. With each exhalation invite the leg to come closer to the chest, and on your inhalation, allow the leg to subtly retract. This subtle oscillation of the leg is supported by the breath and is qualitatively different than "bouncing" during the stretch or pulling on your leg. Stay for at least 1 minute.

Variation B with Hip Turned Outward: Adjust the belt so that it is now wrapped around the *arch* of the right foot. Now turn your right leg outward noting the direction in which your toes are pointing. Draw the right leg in the direction in which the toes are pointing, maintaining the stable position of your pelvis. If the adductors are very tight, don't hesitate to bend the right leg slightly. Simultaneously, draw the left leg into your chest and open the knee out to the left side so that both thighs are at exactly the same angle. Rest your left hand on your left knee and check that the navel is

centered and both buttocks are equally weighted on the floor (Figure 39B). Stay for at least 1 minute.

Variation C with Hip Turned Inward: Return to CRP with the left knee bent and foot firmly on the floor, and the right leg at a 90 degree angle to your trunk. Adjust the belt so that it is now around the *heel* of the foot. Keeping the right leg straight in the air, internally rotate the leg. Slowly draw the leg across the midline of the body keeping both buttocks on the floor. Simultaneously, *internally rotate* the left leg and draw your left knee across the midline keeping the foot on the floor. You will now have both thighs at exactly the same degree of internal rotation, which will help you to keep the pelvis stable. Hold the right end of your yoga belt in your right hand and the left end of the belt in your left hand. Firmly draw downward on the belt until you feel the femur of the right leg anchoring back into the hip socket (Figure 39C). This will further stabilize the pelvis while deepening the sensation of the hip opening. Stay for at least 1 minute and then release back into CRP.

FIGURE 39B

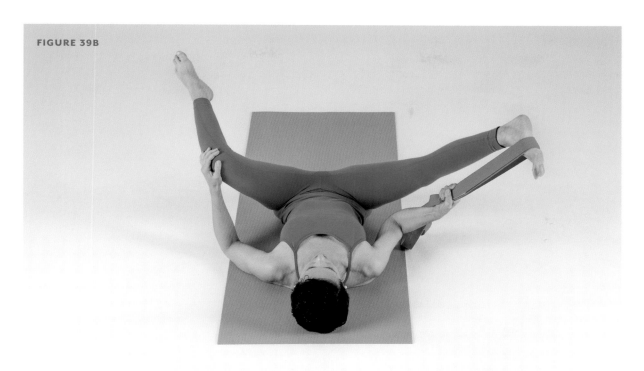

FIGURE 39C

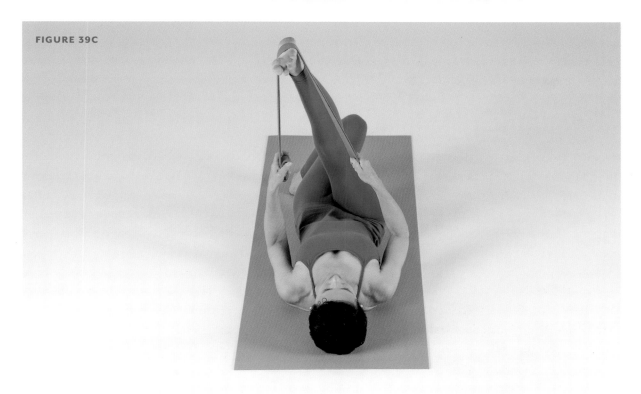

Variation D at the Wall: Lie down in CRP so that your buttocks are about 30 centimeters (1 foot) away from a wall. Bring your left foot up onto the wall so that your leg forms a right angle. Now draw the right leg in toward the chest and turn the knee outward, placing the ankle across

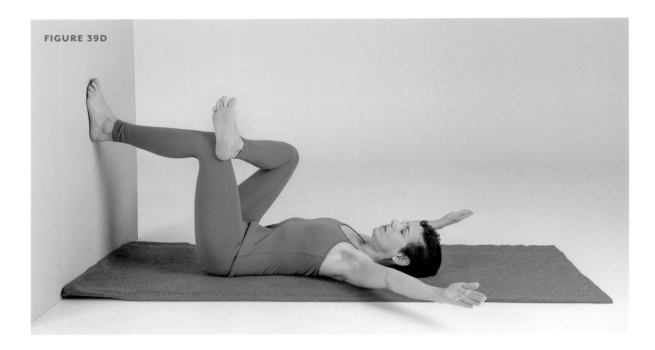

FIGURE 39D

the top of the left thigh. Flex the foot so that the ankle is stable, which will prevent the knee from twisting. Maintain the flexion of the foot as you gently guide the right knee away from your chest toward the wall. Press the left foot firmly into the wall as you continue to stay in the stretch. This is the opening that is required to do Lotus Pose (*Padmasana*), but it must be accomplished without twisting the ankle (supination) so that the external rotation takes place in the hip socket and not in the knee. You can practice this pose with arms down by the sides or with the arms extended diagonally over the head. (Figure 39D). Extending the arms will switch on the core muscles. Stay for at least 1 minute.

Variation E with a Belt: This variation takes a little experimentation, but it can be a fantastic means of feeling your core muscles stabilize your pelvis *while* you open your hips. It is a strong variation, however, so progress to it only after you have comfortably practiced the previous variations. If you have sacroiliac dysfunction or very tight hip flexors, this version may not be suitable for you.

Start in CRP and proceed as in Variation D but without the use of the wall. Make a lasso with your yoga belt so that it wraps around the outside of your right knee, the ball of the left foot, and the sole of your right foot. Keeping your left leg at a right angle, press the left foot into the belt, tightening the belt further so that you feel the right hip opening (Figure 39E). Maintain the perpendicular position of your left leg throughout the movement. Once you have established this position, experiment with bringing your arms out to the sides in line with your shoulders. Raise your arms off the floor. As you do this, you will feel your core muscles engaging more strongly to stabilize the pelvis. If you want an even stronger core engagement, extend your arms diagonally over the head (Figure 39F). Only practice these variations if you can do so without arching through your lower back. Stay for at least 1 minute and then release and begin the whole sequence on your other side.

FIGURE 39E

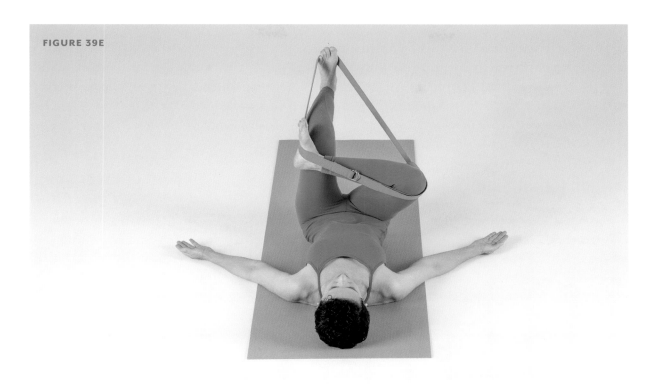

FIGURE 39F

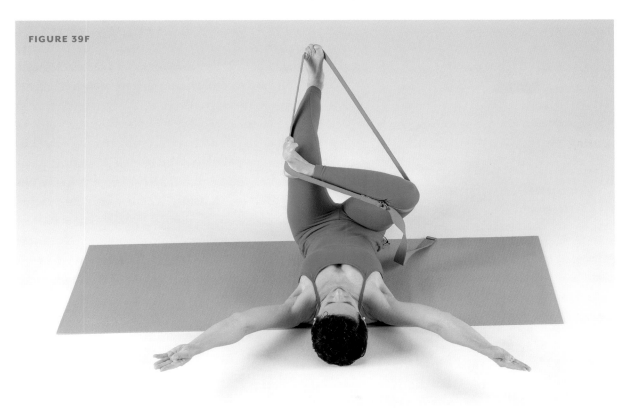

Completion

After any movement that involves extensive hip opening, it's important to do a core stabilization posture. You can practice a few rounds of the Pelvic Reset Adduction, doing the adduction (pressing inward) sequence, with a block between the knees and the feet hip-width apart. Or you can practice several sequential Bridge Poses, starting in CRP with a block between the knees. Slowly lift the tailbone, sacrum, pelvis, and lower back off the floor while keeping T12 on the floor. Then, just as gradually, lengthen and lower the spine back onto the floor.

PRACTICE SUMMARY

- The Pelvic Reset Abduction, Adduction, Alternating Abduction and Adduction
- Supine Big Toe Pose Variation A with Hip Flexion
- Supine Big Toe Pose Variation B with Hip Turned Outward
- Supine Big Toe Pose Variation C with Hip Turned Inward
- Supine Big Toe Pose Variation D at the Wall
- Supine Big Toe Pose Variation E with a Belt
- The Pelvic Reset
- Bridge Pose

❋ *Key Concepts*

▶ Mobility can come at a price—overstretching ligaments can lead to joint instability.

▶ Forcing your hip joints beyond a healthy range of motion can compromise the snug fit between the ilium and sacrum, leading to sacroiliac dysfunction.

▶ Aligning and balancing the bones of the pelvis can alleviate pelvic, low back, and hip pain. Keep your pelvis stable whenever you work on hip mobility.

LIFELONG STRENGTH AND MOBILITY

Getting clear about your core values can be a useful frame of reference for considering the soundness of your Yoga or fitness regimen. Which activities give you pleasure and add meaning to your life? Perhaps you enjoy being able to hike in the mountains, and you'd like to retain this ability well into your senior years. Or you may be an avid gardener, in which case having healthy hips (and knees) will ensure that you can squat or kneel to weed, plant, or harvest. Having a strong lower back will support heftier work, such as shoveling or pushing a laden wheelbarrow, as well as allowing you to play with and pick up grandchildren. In fact, being able to sit comfortably, stand with good posture, lie down for restful sleep, and walk with ease should be the outcome of any balanced Yoga or fitness routine. Sadly, we see people in our classes every day who are no longer able to do many of these basic movements and who live in chronic pain *as a result of* their Yoga practice or so-called fitness routine. This is not the way it is meant to be. Consider whether you are practicing movements right now in your fitness routine that feel forced and uncomfortable. Are these movements worth the risk of compromising your future ability to do important and practical everyday activities?

Rather than living your life so that you can practice Yoga, maintain a balanced wellness routine so that you can live your life. Then, you will reap the benefits of strength, mobility, and ease in your body for many years to come.

CHAPTER 9

Practicing Yoga with Core Awareness

Yoga Sutra II:46: Sthira sukham asanam
"Through steadfastly abiding in the part of the self that is unchanging,
one finds ease within the posture of the moment."
—DONNA FARHI

B Y NOW we hope that you have developed *a felt sense* of your core muscles and are feeling the benefits of softening, lengthening, and strengthening the psoas. Ultimately, this work is about finding your center and being able to do all your everyday activities with ease in your body. When you apply these skills to the practice of Yoga postures or asanas, your awareness will shift from striving toward mobility at all costs to opening the body within the healthy constraint of a strong core.

In this book, we have emphasized the physical dimensions of core balance, but we also have offered a more encompassing definition of what it means to be truly centered. It's likely that having experienced many of the physical practices, you are starting to notice that centering your body can facilitate changes to your energetic, emotional, mental, and even spiritual state of being.

INTEGRATION AND TRANSFORMATION

A central concept within the Yoga tradition is the ethical precept of *yama* (to yoke or restrain). This term usually is related to ethical practices, such as not stealing or not harming, but it also can be used to infer a deeper meaning to the physical practices. When the practice of *yama* is employed during asana, the emphasis of each practice is on maintaining *stillness* and *stability* while in movement. For many practitioners, this is a radical reversal of focus. Rather than the practice being driven by a mind exclusively future-focused on "how far and how much," attention instead is placed on the present moment and on maintaining stability.

143

As you move, attention remains fixed on the *non-moving* support of the movement. When you practice in this way, something extraordinary happens: the mind becomes still, the breath becomes even, and the emotions (whatever they may be) begin to settle. Practicing in this way cultivates a unity between the mind and body, one of the definitions of Yoga itself.

In the many years that we have shared with our students this Yogic approach to core balance, three general themes of transformation have emerged. First, and most common, students report transformation toward a state of feeling more *grounded*, *connected*, and *supported*. Accessing a secure relationship with the ground (*Sthira: the Yogic principal of steadiness*) can generate a kinesthetic experience of being seated in the self—trusting yourself, trusting life, and feeling comfortable in your own skin. In this state of groundedness, peacefulness and ease (*Sukha: the Yogic principle of relaxation*) are much more accessible. Many students have learned to contact a deep stillness that lies within their energetic core and return to it deliberately and intentionally.

Second, students report transformation toward a state of *self-support* and *self-regulation*. When you have a clear sense of your own center of gravity, you remain in touch with your own needs. You are less likely to be easily swayed by others or to look for external validation. This self-reliance gives you a powerful base from which to *respond* rather than *react* to changing circumstances. Your increased capacity for responsiveness creates resilience and the ability to more quickly bounce back from challenging events.

Third, students report transformation toward a state of being *present in the moment*. When your body is off center, it is more difficult to be present with *what is*, partly because your nervous system is preoccupied with trying to prevent you from losing balance. When you focus on centering your physical body, the mind begins to relinquish its

infatuation with planning and worrying about the future. Instead of wrestling with how things should be, you become more able to see things just as they are. Paradoxically, this ability to be present with things just as they are provides the perfect footing to be able to move skillfully forward toward a higher purpose or vision for your life.

These three themes—being grounded, being self-reliant, and being present—are interrelated and often are experienced simultaneously to one degree or another. Although you initially may work with core balancing to soothe physical discomfort, the physical healing can ignite a journey toward integration, congruence, and wholeness. What began as a physical exploration can lead to a transformative journey from disempowerment toward personal authority, from compensations toward authenticity, and from the tyranny of the ego toward a compassionate presence.

In the Yoga asanas presented in this chapter, we will suggest some points of focus that will help you keep your core stable as you explore mobilizing and opening your body. Because the psoas muscle is the keystone within the Cylinder of Support, we'll frequently refer back to this muscle, asking you to practice some or all of the following:

- Stabilize the origin or the insertion (the spine or the femur)
- Move one end of the muscle (the spine or the femur) away from the stabilized end
- Condense (move the two ends of the muscle together)
- Lengthen (move the two ends of the muscle apart)

When you intentionally focus your mind on the deep core psoas muscles and visualize them changing shape as you move, the quality of your movement changes. Using visual imagery to evoke changes to your alignment and movement

❖ Emotional Transformation

Our students consistently have reported the following transformations:

Aggression	*toward*	Assertion
Disempowerment	*toward*	Empowerment
Fragility	*toward*	Robustness
Emotional Confusion	*toward*	Emotional Congruence
Bravado	*toward*	Vulnerability
Fear	*toward*	Trust
Inability to Love	*toward*	Opening to Love
Rigidity	*toward*	Fluidity
Self-Criticism	*toward*	Self-Acceptance
Suppression	*toward*	Expression
Weakness	*toward*	Strength
Victimhood	*toward*	Ownership

has the same effect. Mindfully softening, lengthening, condensing, or moving from your psoas overrides habitual ways of moving. This focused attention can be used to establish safer and more efficient neural pathways. It also provides an internal focus that can steady your mind. In Yogic language, directing your attention to a specific place in the body is known as a *drishti* point. Remember that when you consciously activate the psoas first, the other core muscles follow suit.

As you experiment with the postures, observe how you establish and maintain your stability as you move. The previous steps in the protocol have given you the skills to make conscious decisions about how to use the psoas muscles in different types of movements. Notice when, where, and how you "lose it." For instance you may have a habit of overarching your lower back or jutting your rib cage; both are signs that you have lost the anchoring support of the origin of the psoas. Or you may have a habit of losing the neutral position of your pelvis, which is a sign you have lost the anchoring support of the insertion of the psoas. As you become aware of your own particular habits, notice whether a steady focus on the psoas muscles, the visualization of the Figure-8 Loop (Chapter Seven, pages 115–117), or some of the other images we have suggested can assist you. If your own images and ideas spontaneously appear, that is even better.

❖❖ INQUIRIES: *Engaging Your Psoas*

Engaging the psoas can be defined as the conscious skill of *simultaneously* creating both gentle positive tension *and* elongation between the two ends of the psoas muscle. Remember all the psoas muscle bundles with their overlapping attachments and various angles of pull? During any movement, some psoas muscle bundles are working in the capacity of "movers," while others are working in the capacity of "stabilizers." And remember that the viscoelastic quality of psoas fascia creates a resistance to both contraction and elongation, maintaining a stiffness or *pullback* in the tissue throughout a movement. This viscoelasticity creates *cohesion* as the psoas is contracting and *applies the brakes* on elongation. These healthy *yamas* or constraints make movement safer and more deliberate. ❖❖

❖❖ *Engaging Your Psoas during Forward Bending*

Stand with your feet hip-width apart. Now step your left leg back so that your feet are about 1 meter (3 feet) apart. Turn your left foot 45 degrees outward while keeping your hips square. Place

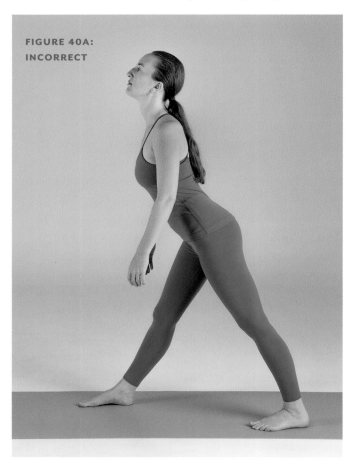

FIGURE 40A: INCORRECT

your hands on the general location of the psoas muscles. Now slowly bend forward from your hips keeping your spine straight. Come forward 20 degrees off the vertical and pause. Imagine that you are sending strong anchors down from each psoas muscle to the ground. Feel the left and right psoas muscles like strong yet pliant pillars supporting your lumbar spine. Some students like to imagine the psoas muscles as hands lifting and supporting the front of the spine. Now come forward another 20 degrees, pausing to check that you are not collapsing at the juncture between the pelvis and lumbar spine (S1/L5), or between the lumbar spine and the ribcage (L5/T12) (Figure 40A, incorrect). Each time you move incrementally, reestablish the anchors from the psoas to the ground. If your core muscles are weak, you may only be able to come forward about 45 degrees without compensating or losing your anchor. Eventually, you may be able to come to an approximate tabletop position (Figure 40B). Maintain this position for five breaths. To come out of the posture, bend your right knee and slowly push down into the floor to bring your torso back to the starting position. Visualize the psoas muscles supporting and lifting your spine back to the upright position. When practiced correctly, you will feel that you are elongating through your spine while simultaneously creating a slight braking action to that very same elongation. ⁞

THE YOGA POSTURES

The Yoga postures that follow are intended to heighten your awareness of psoas integration and core stability within your practice. This chapter is not intended to be a comprehensive how-to guide to Yoga.[1] We have put together a sampling of postures that are particularly helpful for developing a balanced psoas and a strong core body. As you practice these poses, incorporate the learning from each step of the protocol. To make a pose into a *psoas event*, consciously use the appropriate imagery to help you elongate, condense, or move from the psoas. To focus your awareness, it may be helpful initially to practice poses placing your hands on the psoas attachments. Experiment with different core visualizations to determine which ones give you the most stability. The postures can be done as a sequence, or they can be inserted individually into your existing movement routine. You can apply what you learn from these practices to other Yoga postures and movement practices.

At the end of this chapter, you will find some handy practice sequences that incorporate tech-

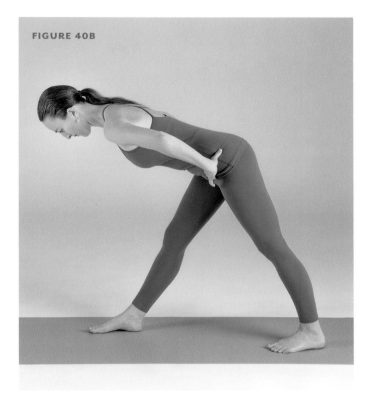

FIGURE 40B

niques from other chapters in this book. Many of the psoas releases require that you stay in the pose for at least 5 minutes. We highly recommend using a smart phone app to create interval timings, so that you can relax into the practices with the assurance that you are giving your right and left sides equal attention. Enjoy!

PRACTICES

Simple Warrior Pose I (*Virabhadrasana I*)

Benefits
- Provides an easy way to feel your psoas muscles at the beginning of your Yoga practice.
- Gently opens the groin.
- Elongates the spine.

Contraindications
- None.

You'll Need
- A yoga mat and bare feet.

Why: Because the psoas muscles are buried deep within the body, it can be helpful to touch base with these muscles at the beginning of a Yoga practice, Pilates routine, or other exercise regimen. This practice is a fantastic prelude to other "lunge" practices.

How: Stand with your feet together and slowly turn your right foot outward about 45 degrees. On an inhalation, extend both your arms over your head (Figure 41A). Feel the sensation along the right groin and observe whether you also can feel a connection up the right side of the lumbar spine. Reaching the arms slightly off-center to the left may intensify the sensation (Figure 41B). After a few breaths bring your arms down by your sides and repeat the exercise on your left side.

Points of Focus (for the right side)

- Anchor both psoas muscles all the way down the legs to the ground.
- As you take your arms over your head, stabilize the solar plexus area to prevent the lower rib cage from jutting forward.

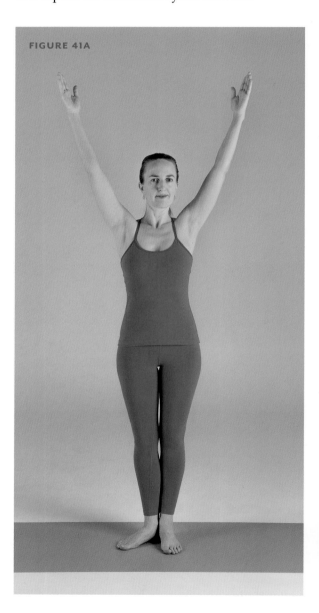

FIGURE 41A

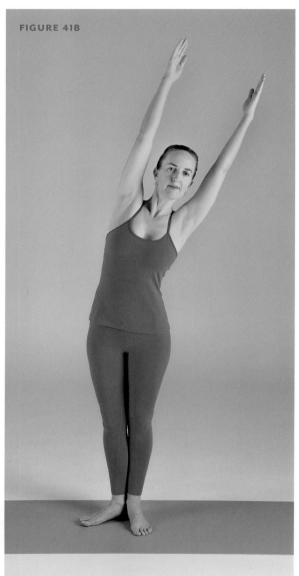

FIGURE 41B

Horseman's Pose (*Utkatasana*)

Benefits
- Strengthens the thighs, abdominal muscles, and spine.
- Warms the body and improves endurance.

Contraindications
- People with chronic hip, knee, or ankle pain should practice with caution.

You'll Need
- A yoga mat.

Why: Horseman's Pose can be added to almost any Yoga practice routine to improve core strength. It is an ideal addition at the beginning of the Sun Salutation (*Suryanamaskar*).

How: Stand with the inner edges of your feet touching. This will help you to engage your adductors (inner thigh muscles). On an inhalation, extend your arms overhead and hook your thumbs. Reaching strongly upward, slowly bend your knees. As you deepen in the position, maintain a clear line from your head through to your tailbone (Figure 42A). Do not deepen your squat

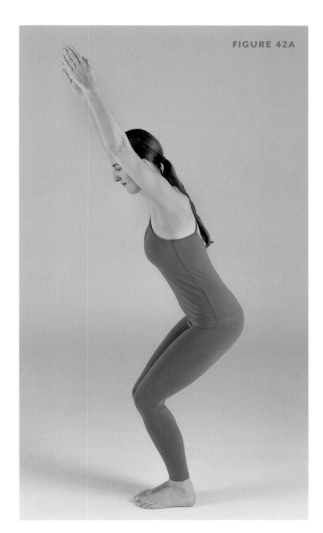

FIGURE 42A

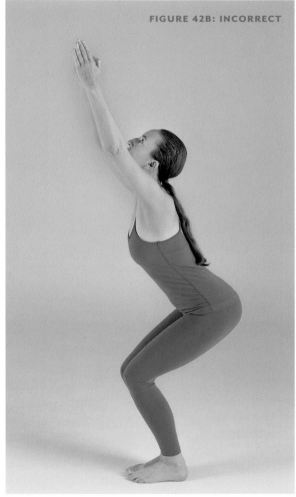

FIGURE 42B: INCORRECT

if this results in an accentuation of your lumbar curve (Figure 42B, incorrect). Arching the neck and looking upward will tend to accentuate the lumbar curve, whereas keeping your gaze neutral or even looking slightly downward can facilitate greater stability throughout the lower back. Stay here for three to five breaths and then slowly release, coming back to a standing position.

Points of Focus

- Stabilize the solar plexus area to prevent hinging through the base of the rib cage.
- Keep the Cylinder of Support switched on by engaging the Figure-8 Loop (see pages 115–117).
- Feel the left and right psoas muscles becoming long and lean as they support the front of the spine.

Warrior Pose II (*Virabhadrasana II*)

Benefits

- Strengthens the legs and increases the flexibility of the hips and groin.
- Warms the body.
- Increases stamina and determination.

Contraindications

- People with cardiac problems or high blood pressure should approach this pose with caution. To reduce strain on the heart, practice this posture with the arms down by your sides, hands on hips.

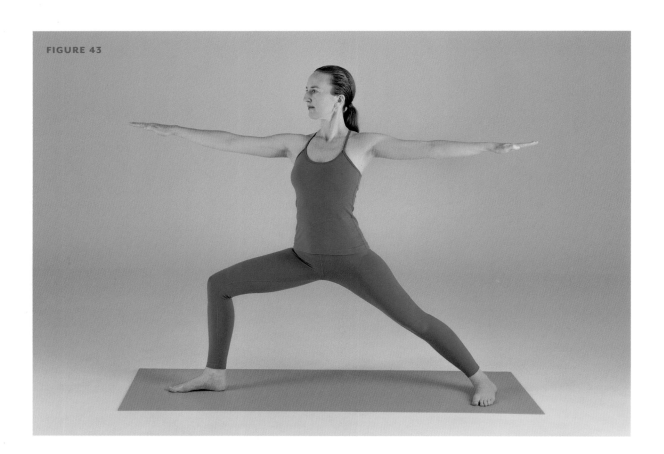

FIGURE 43

You'll Need
- A yoga mat.

Why: This is one of the safest and most effective Yoga postures for opening the psoas. Because the spine is in a relatively neutral position, this is a particularly safe practice for people with back problems.

How: Stand with the feet wide apart so that your feet are positioned under your wrists when the arms are extended. This is an approximate distance—adapt according to your body proportions. Turn both feet about 30 degrees inward so that the knees can align over your ankles. As you breathe in, expand your arms out to the sides. Now turn the right foot and leg 90 degrees outward. On an exhalation, slowly bend your right knee several inches. Without coming up, push horizontally back through your right leg until you can feel the weight coming into your back foot. Eventually your front thigh will be parallel to the floor (Figure 43).

Allow the left side of the pelvis to come slightly forward so that the right knee can align directly over the right foot. For the safety of your knee joints, this alignment is absolutely non-negotiable. Keeping this in mind, see how much you can open the left groin without compromising the alignment of your front leg. When practiced correctly, you will feel a strong opening in your left groin. Stay for three to thirteen breaths (depending on your current level of conditioning), and then return to your preparatory stance, resting your arms down by your sides. Now practice the posture on the left side.

Points of Focus (for the right side)
- Observe whether the pelvis tips anteriorly over the right thigh. Explore condensing the right psoas and lengthening the left psoas to balance the pelvis.
- Note whether the space between the sternum and the pubic bone has increased so that the abdomen is falling forward. Condense the upper psoas and engage the Cylinder of Support to bring the pelvis back into a neutral position.
- Visualize sending an anchor down both psoas muscles to the ground.

Warrior I Flow Sequence (*Virabhadrasana I Vinyasana*)

Benefits
- Opens the front of the groin releasing the deep psoas muscles.
- Strengthens the legs and spinal muscles.
- Reduces kyphosis (excessive thoracic curvature).

Contraindications
- People with heart conditions or high blood pressure should be cautious if this sequence causes strain. If you have very weak core and back muscles, do this variation with your arms either reaching out to the side (like an airplane) or reaching back toward your hips.

You'll Need
- A yoga mat.
- A chair or yoga block (if you have tight hamstrings).

Why: This is an excellent practice to counter the effects of long periods of sitting. It not only lengthens the psoas muscles, it also opens the shoulders and strengthens the upper back to support erect posture.

How: Stand with your feet hip-width apart. Imagine that you are standing on two railway tracks. Keep your left leg on the track as you step the foot behind you, turning the left foot about 20 degrees outward. The feet will be 1 meter or so (3–4 feet) apart. If your stance is too deep, the left side of the pelvis will be twisted. Adjust your feet so that the pelvis is even to the front of the room. As you inhale extend both arms over your head, with the palms facing forward (Figure 44A). As you exhale, slowly bend the right knee, keeping the abdomen upright (Figure 44B). As you inhale, bend both elbows to form a square and slightly tilt your lower arms about 20 degrees backward (Figure 44C). This is a *tiny* movement that targets the upper back muscles—don't make the mistake of extending the arms behind you and arching your lower back (Figure 44D, incorrect). It's important to keep your core body and lumbar spine in a

neutral position so that the deeper opening of the psoas can occur.

Now as you exhale, hinge forward from your hips while slowly extending your arms in front of you until your spine is almost parallel to the floor. Keep your front leg bent (Figure 44E). If having your arms extended over the head causes strain on your back, you can either extend the arms to the side or you can extend the arms back so that your hands rest against your hips. Take a breath in and hold while in this position. As you exhale, slowly straighten the front leg and place both hands on the floor (or on a yoga block or chair, depending on your flexibility; Figure 44F). Take one breath in and out. On your next breath in, slowly bend your front leg and push down through your front foot to support your ascent back up into Warrior I

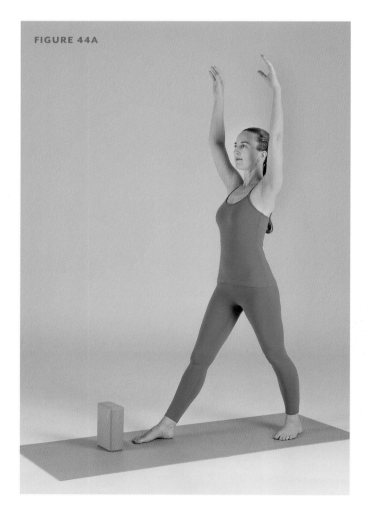

FIGURE 44A

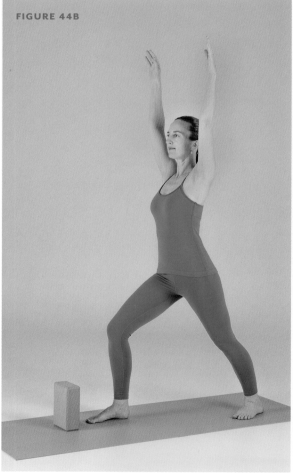

FIGURE 44B

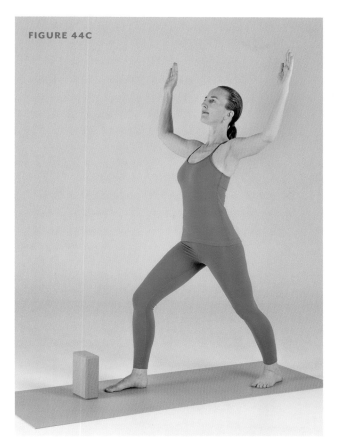

FIGURE 44C

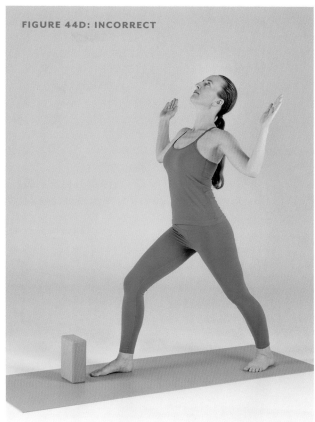

FIGURE 44D: INCORRECT

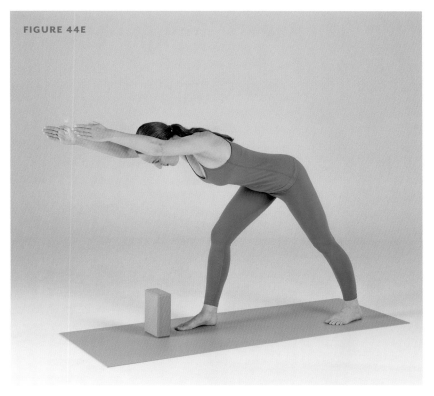

FIGURE 44E

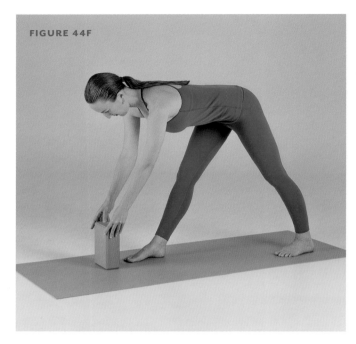

FIGURE 44F

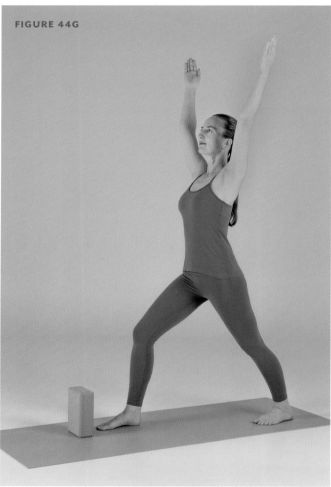

FIGURE 44G

(Figure 44G). Extend your arms either out to the sides or over your head, on a full inhalation, and return the arms back down to your sides as you exhale. Repeat this cycle another two or three times and then practice the sequence on your left side.

Points of Focus

- Bring your attention to T12 at the base of your rib cage. Keep this point stable throughout the whole sequence.
- Keep the pelvis in a neutral position, engaging the Cylinder of Support to give your spine optimal support throughout the movement. This will ensure that you eccentrically lengthen the psoas, rather than hinging on your lumbar spine.
- Visualize the dynamic tension created as the arms pull the upper psoas into elongation while the lower psoas is anchored down the legs to the ground.

Half Reclining Hero's Pose (*Ardha Supta Virasana*)

Benefits

- Provides an intensive release of the quadriceps, paving the way to access the psoas and iliacus.
- Helps to correct hyperlordosis.

Contraindications

- The following variations of Hero's Pose can be difficult for people with knee injuries. Raise your pelvis as high as you require for comfort. If sitting on a bolster while kneeling still creates discomfort in your knee joints, these variations may not be suitable for you.

You'll Need

- A yoga mat covered with a blanket.
- One to three blankets to raise the pelvis.
- Two firm bolsters.

Why: All of the following variations of Hero's Pose create an intensive stretch of the quadriceps (the flexor muscles on the front of the thigh) and also address tightness in the psoas muscles. If you are a runner or athlete and have developed tightness in your quadriceps, you will find that you have to release the quadriceps before you can gain access to the deeper musculature of the psoas.

How: Usually, Reclining Hero's Pose is practiced with both thighs together (knees flexed, hips extended), which can put an enormous pull on the insertion of the psoas at the hip as well as the origin of the psoas in the lower back. It's not surprising that one of the most common complaints in this pose is a feeling of "pinching" and compression in the lumbar spine. This feeling likely is caused by tightness in the lower fibers of the psoas pulling the lumbar spine forward into hyperextension (see Illustration 6B, page 15). By practicing with one leg bent in Hero's Pose and the other leg either extended straight or flexed, one has optimal control over the pelvis. By keeping the pelvis in a neutral or slightly posteriorly rotated position (tucked under), the psoas essentially is forced to lengthen rather than contract, and best of all, there should be no sense of compression or pain in the lower back. Our personal experience of this sequence is that it not only lengthens the psoas but also can correct long-standing torques and rotations of the pelvis that may contribute to sacroiliac dysfunction. Practice each position for 3 minutes. (It is useful to have a timer to ensure that you give equal time to both sides.)

Variation A with Leg Extended: Place two bolsters in a T-shape formation behind you so that you can recline back at an angle. Sit in Hero's Pose with the buttocks raised on a folded blanket or bolster to ensure that both knees are comfortable. In this kneeling position, the tops of your feet will rest close to the sides of your hips. Check that the inner and outer corners of the kneecap are equidistant to the floor and that the thighs are parallel to each other. The center of the knee should be in line with the center of the femur. In this position, there will be a little space between the thighs. Slowly release the right leg and strongly extend this leg from the back of the waist to the heel. Check that your pelvis is level and, if necessary, place a folded blanket under the right buttock. Carefully lower yourself onto the bolster. Draw the pubic bone toward the navel, pressing the shin of the left leg into the floor to activate a sense of lifting and reaching from the tail (Figure 45A). If your quadriceps muscles are tight, you may feel this posture primarily in the muscles of your left thigh. Once the quadriceps is sufficiently released (which can take weeks or months . . .) you will feel the opening deep in the groin and lower psoas. Stay for 3 minutes and then change to the other side.

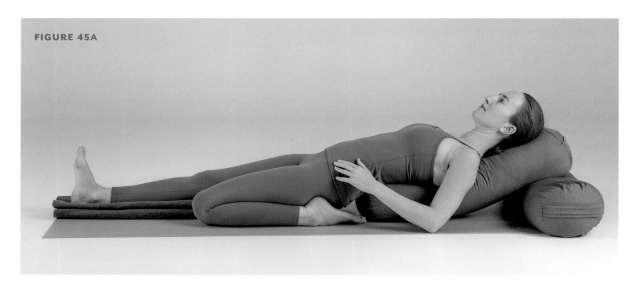

FIGURE 45A

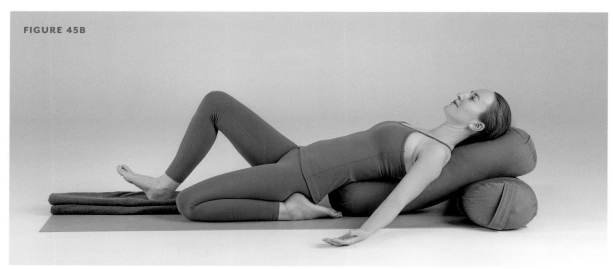

FIGURE 45B

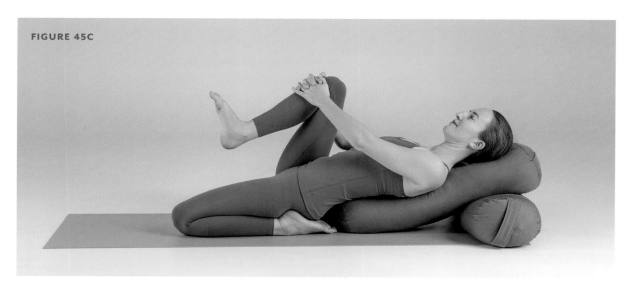

FIGURE 45C

Variation B with One Leg Bent: Assume Hero's Pose as in Variation A with the same propping. Now bring the right leg forward with the knee bent and the ankle flexed. Press firmly into the right heel to encourage the pelvis to move into a neutral or slightly posteriorly rotated position (Figure 45B). Stay for 3 minutes and then change to the other side.

Variation C with Knee to Chest: This strong variation is not for everyone. If it feels too intense, simply repeat Variation B. To begin, assume Hero's Pose as in Variation A with the same propping. Next, bend the right leg and draw the knee in toward the chest, firmly grasping the leg around the shin. This draws the pelvis into an even stronger position of flexion (Figure 45C). Stay for 3 minutes and then change to the other side.

When you complete this series, you may wish to practice Reclining Hero's Pose with both legs together. Many people who previously felt compression and pain in the lower back are delighted to discover that the lower back is now more likely to be pain free. Keep in mind that Reclining Hero's Pose is not meant to be a back bend. As much as is possible, the spine should be in a neutral position and the opening should occur deep in the thigh and groin. If the lower back is deeply arched, raise your back onto a bolster until you achieve a sense of ease in the knees and spine. Only attempt coming down onto the floor if you can do so without discomfort.

Points of Focus
- Draw the tail toward the pubic bone to keep the pelvis in a neutral position.
- Simultaneously stabilize the upper attachments at the solar plexus and visualize cohesion between the two ends of the psoas.

Gateway Pose (*Parighasana*)

Benefits
- Improves breathing by stretching rib muscles.
- Lengthens the side body.
- Strengthens the core muscles.

Contraindications
- People with knee or hip injury should be cautious.

You'll Need
- A yoga mat.
- A yoga blanket to cushion your knees.

Why: Often Gateway Pose is done as a side bending movement of the spine. This variation focuses on maintaining length in both psoas muscles throughout the pose. This allows the spine to remain aligned while the pelvis hinges sideways over the leg. In this way, the lateral movement of the spine is permitted only as the psoas lengthens. This rendition of the pose may not be as glorious, but the psoas muscles get a good workout.

How: Kneel on the floor so the pelvis is directly above the knees. Extend the right leg sideways ensuring that the left hip remains stacked above the left knee. Turn the right foot outward and extend the toes toward the floor. Place the hands on the left psoas attachments. With successive exhalations, hinge the pelvis sideways over the straight leg (Figure 46A). Move in small

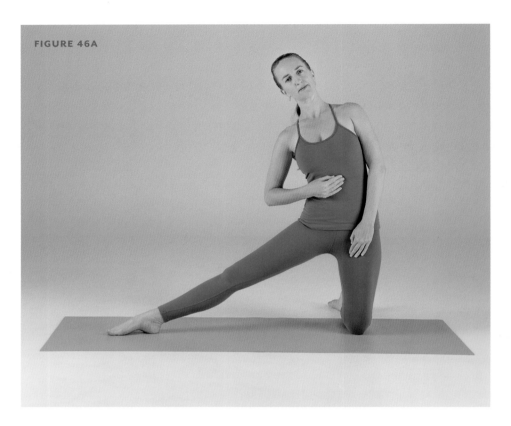

FIGURE 46A

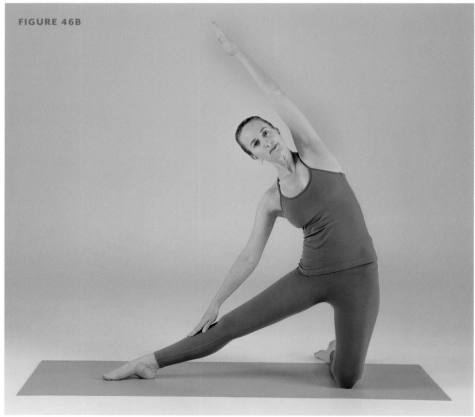

FIGURE 46B

increments, taking several breaths to complete the movement. As soon as the spine begins to side bend, return to the upright position on an inhalation. Fold the right leg back into a kneeling position and repeat the pose on the other side. Once you get the somatic sensation of lengthening the psoas, you can repeat the pose with the left arm overhead reaching toward the extended leg, and the right hand resting on the straight leg (Figure 46B).

Points of Focus (for the right side)

- Send an anchor down the left psoas all the way to the ground.
- Visualize the left psoas lengthening and allowing the spine to move laterally.
- When doing the pose with the arm overhead, visualize the arm pulling the upper psoas into greater length.

Downward Facing Dog (*Adho Mukha Svanasana*)

Benefits

- Elongates and releases tension throughout the entire spinal column.
- Stretches the hamstrings and Achilles tendons.
- Strengthens the wrists, arms, and shoulders.

Contraindications

- People with carpal tunnel syndrome or injuries to the wrists should be cautious.
- People with high blood pressure, glaucoma, or detached retina should not practice this pose.

- Those with recent disk injuries should start with Half Downward Facing Dog Pose (*Ardha Adho Mukha Svanasana*; page 103).

You'll Need

- A yoga mat.

Why: Downward Facing Dog is one of the most versatile of all the Yoga postures. It is also a posture in which we commonly see people overarching

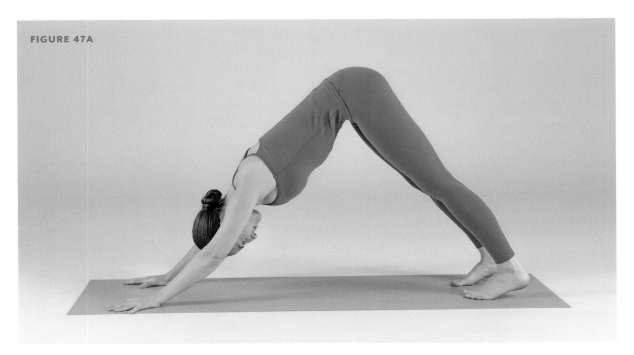

FIGURE 47A

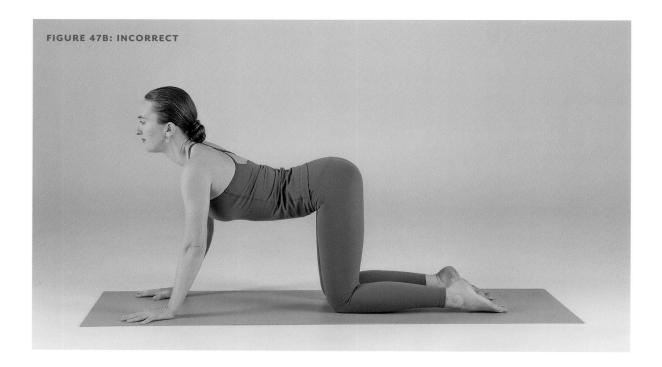

FIGURE 47B: INCORRECT

the back (destabilizing the spine and core) in the false belief that this action lengthens the spine. Learning to elongate rather than extend the back is a foundation skill for all other practices.

How: Come onto all-fours with the spine in a neutral position. Take a breath in, and then as you breathe out, push back through your arms lifting your pelvis up and back as you straighten your legs (Figure 47A). Maintain the neutral spinal curves as you elongate the spine on successive exhalations. Take a peek down the front of your body. If your lower ribs are jutting forward, you probably are bridging your mid-spine and hyper-extending your back. We find that people often begin in a collapsed all-fours position and then carry this hyperextension into their Downward Facing Dog Pose (Figure 47B, incorrect). Practice

some of the Points of Focus to reestablish your neutral spine when on all-fours and sustain this as you push back into the posture. Stay for three to thirteen breaths, coming down on an exhalation and resting in Child's Pose (*Balasana*). Practice twice more, resting in between repetitions.

Points of Focus

- Move the sternum back into the body. This will help you to stabilize through the origin of the psoas at T12.
- Feel the left and right psoas muscles streaming along the length of the lumbar spine and providing support.
- Imagine casting an anchor from T12 around the two sides of the pelvis, all the way down the backs of both legs to the heels. This will help to stabilize your lower back.

Sage Pose (*Bharadvajasana*)

Benefits
- Releases the hips and lower back.
- Opens the shoulders, chest, and lungs.

Contraindications
- People with disk injuries should be cautious.

You'll Need
- A yoga mat and two blankets.

Why: Twists release the deep intervertebral muscles (the tiny muscles between the vertebrae of the spine) and can be wonderful counter postures to forward bends and back bends.

How: Kneel on a blanket and slowly let your hips slide off your heels until you are sitting to the right of your feet. Place a folded blanket underneath your right buttock until both sides of your pelvis are level. As you inhale, anchor your weight through the surfaces of your body that are in contact with the floor, and as you exhale, slowly turn to the right, bringing your left hand onto the outside of your right knee (Figure 48). Use your right hand just behind your right buttock to help maintain the lift through your back. Stay for 1 minute and then slowly release and repeat on the second side.

Points of Focus (*for the right side*)
- Before you twist to the right, anchor the insertions of both psoas muscles.
- As you twist to the right, visualize both psoas muscles lengthening.

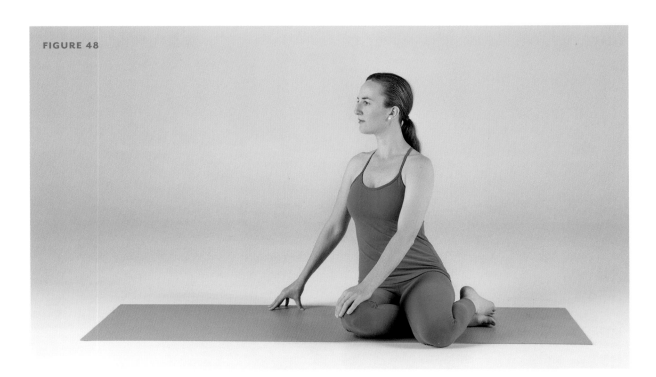

FIGURE 48

Corpse Pose (*Savasana*)

Benefits
- Calms and relaxes the entire body.
- Provides a time to digest and assimilate all previous practices.

Contraindications
- None.

You'll Need
- A yoga mat and a blanket.
- Bolsters and a bath towel.

Why: Before beginning any practice we've encouraged you to do a Body Weather Reading (see pages 6–7) to gauge how you are feeling. At the end of your practice, it is just as important to notice any positive changes that have occurred as a result of your practice. Relaxation allows those positive changes "to land" in your body.

How: Lie on a yoga mat cushioned with a blanket. Place a bolster underneath your lower thighs and knees. If your heels are not firmly in contact with the ground, support them with a bath towel. Similarly, if your head tends to arch back, place a folded bath towel or blanket underneath your neck and head until the back of the skull rests easily on the floor (Figure 49). Stay here for 5–20 minutes. Make a habit of noticing at least one positive change that has occurred as a result of your practice.

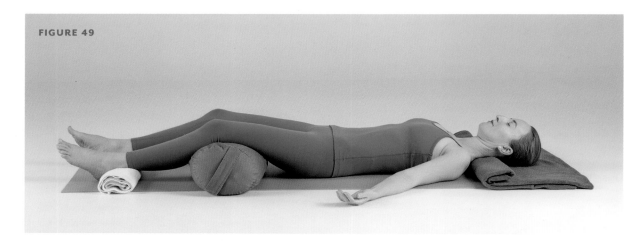

FIGURE 49

Points of Focus
- Focus on the anchor point of T12 (the base of the kidneys). As you exhale, lengthen from this point all the way through the back of the body down to your heels.
- With each exhalation, imagine the base of the rib cage releasing away from the top rim of the pelvis.
- With successive exhalations, visualize the psoas softening and nestling along both sides of the spine.

Practice Sequence A: Building Strength
Physical Effect: Strengthens core muscles and centers the mind.
Energetic Effect: Stimulates and improves stamina.
Practice Time: 30 minutes

1. The *WHO* Breath
   (1–3 rounds of 10 breaths;
   1–4 minutes) . . . . **(PAGE 45)**

2. Low Bridge Pose
   (*Setu Bandhasana*)
   (×8, 5 minutes) . . . . **(PAGE 125)**

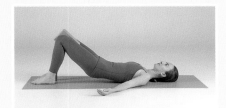

3. Dynamic Bridge
   (*Setu Bandhasana*)
   (×3, 5 minutes) . . . . **(PAGE 126)**

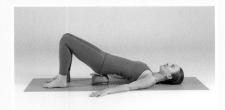

4. Heel and Toe Touches
   (1–3 minutes) . . . . **(PAGE 124)**

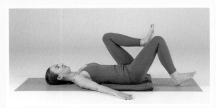

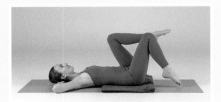

5. Drawing Circles
   (1–3 minutes) . . . . **(PAGE 128)**

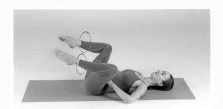

6. Pelvic Reset (5 minutes) . . . . . **(PAGES 133–137)**

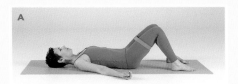

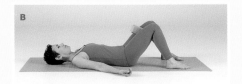

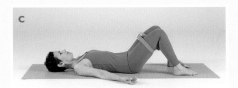

7. Corpse Pose (*Savasana*)
   (5–10 minutes) . . . . **(PAGE 162)**

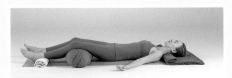

Practice Sequence B: Core Yoga Basics
Physical Effect: Builds core strength, releases the psoas, and opens the upper back.
Energetic Effect: Exhilarates and warms.
Practice Time: 30–45 minutes

1. Simple Warrior Pose I (*Virabhadrasana I*)
(30 seconds each side) . . . . **(PAGE 147)**

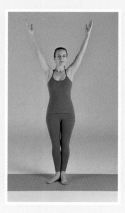

2. Horseman's Pose (*Utkatasana*)
(×3, 15–30 seconds) . . . . **(PAGE 149)**

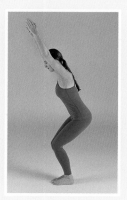

3. Warrior Pose II (*Virabhadrasana II*)
(×2 each side, 15 seconds–1 minute) . **(PAGE 150)**

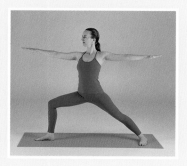

4. Warrior I Flow Sequence
(*Virabhadrasana I Vinyasana*)
(×3 each side) . . . . **(PAGES 151–154)**

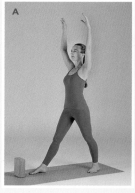
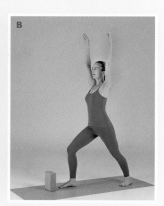
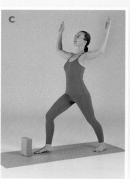
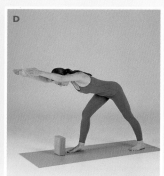
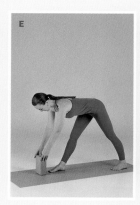
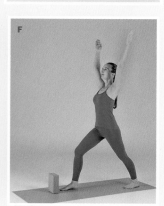

sequence continues on next page ⟶

5. Gateway Pose (*Parighasana*)
(×1 each side, 30 seconds–1 minute) . .

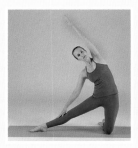

6. Half Reclining Hero's Pose
(*Ardha Supta Virasana*)
(×3, 3 minutes each side) . . . .

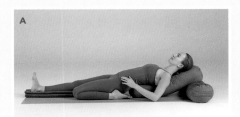

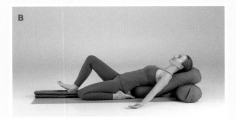

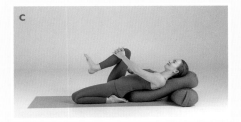

7. Downward Facing Dog
(*Adho Mukha Svanasana*)
(×3, 30 seconds–1 minute) . . . . . .

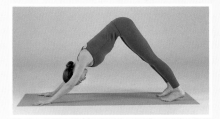

8. Sage Pose One (*Bharadvajasana I*)
(1 minute each side) . . . .

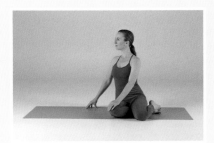

9. Corpse Pose (*Savasana*)
(5–15 minutes) . . . .

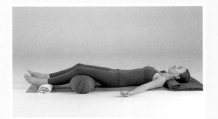

Practice Sequence C: Building Flexibility

Physical Effect: Increases hip and general spinal mobility.

Energetic Effect: Relaxes and rejuvenates.

Practice Time: 45–60 minutes

1. Hydrating the Psoas and
   Spinal Muscles (10 minutes) . . . **(PAGES 60–64)**

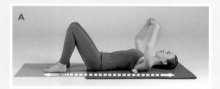

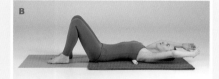

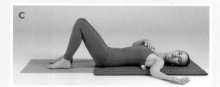

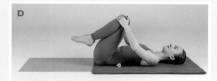

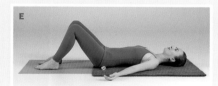

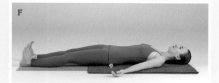

2. Supine Big Toe Pose
   (*Supta Padangusthasana*)
   (5 minutes each side) . . . . **(PAGES 137–141)**

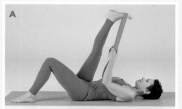
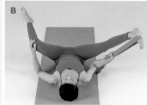

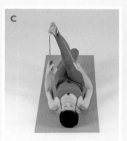
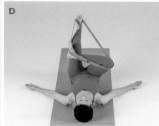

3. Low Bridge Pose
   (*Setu Bandhasana*)
   ×8, 5 minutes) . . . . **(PAGE 125)**

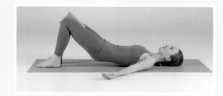

4. Half Supine Hero's Pose
   (*Ardha Supta Virasana*)
   (3 minutes each side) . . . . **(PAGE 157)**

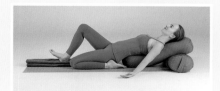

sequence continues on next page ⟶

5. Downward Facing Dog
(*Adho Mukha Svanasana*)
(×3, 30 seconds–1 minute) . . . . . **(PAGE 159)**

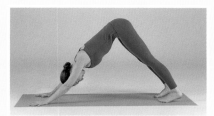

6. Upward Puppy Spiral
(×7 each side, 5–7 minutes) . . . **(PAGES 67–71)**

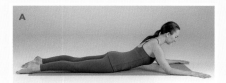

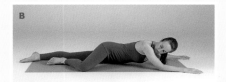

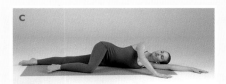

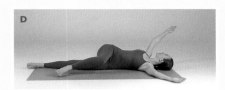

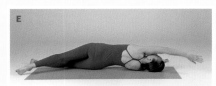

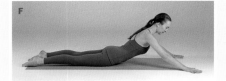

7. Cobra Pose
Variation A, B, or C
(×3, 30 seconds–1 minute) . . . . . **(PAGE 83)**

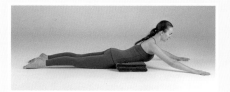

8. Child's Pose
(*Balasana*)
(1 minute) . . . . **(PAGE 84)**

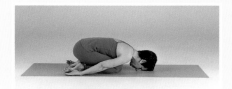

9. The Great Rejuvenator
(*Viparita Karani*)
(5–10 minutes) . . . . **(PAGES 129–130)**

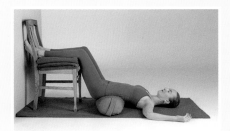

10. Corpse Pose
(*Savasana*)
(5–10 minutes) . . . . **(PAGES 162)**

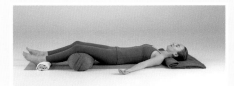

Practice Sequence D: Office Workers' Spinal Recovery

Physical Effect: Releases the spine after long hours of sitting.
Energetic Effect: Soothes and calms.
Practice Time: 30–40 minutes

1. Constructive Rest Position,
   Variation A with MR Ball[2]
   (10 minutes) . . . . **(PAGE 48)**

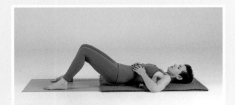

2. Prone Half-Butterfly with MR Ball
   (7 minutes each side) . . . . **(PAGE 64)**

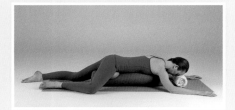

3. Half-Bow with Isometric Releases
   (*Ardha Dhanurasana*)
   (×5 each side, 5 minutes) . . . . **(PAGE 78)**

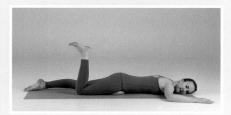

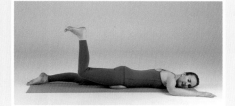

4. Downward Facing Dog
   (*Adho Mukha Svanasana*)
   (×3, 30 seconds–1 minute) . . . . . . **(PAGE 159)**

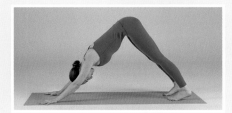

5. Therapeutic Psoas Release
   (5 minutes) . . . . **(PAGE 86)**

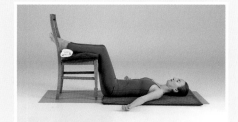

Practice Sequence E: The Decompression Series

Physical Effect: Hydrates, loosens, and releases deep tension in the spinal muscles. Excellent after a long drive or long-haul flight.

Energetic Effect: Energizes and lightens.

Practice Time: 30 minutes

1. Hydrating the Psoas and Spinal Muscles
   (10 minutes) . . . . (PAGES 60–64)

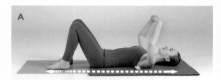

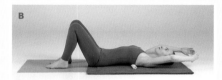

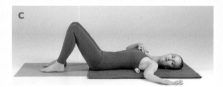

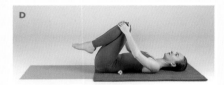

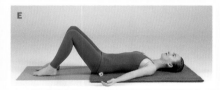

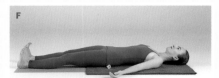

2. Supine Big Toe Pose
   (*Supta Padangusthasana*)
   (5 minutes each side) . . . . . . (PAGES 137–141)

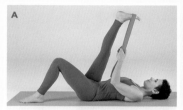
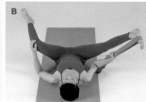
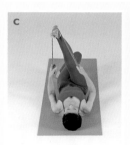
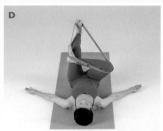

3. Releasing the Psoas on a Bolster
   (1 minute each side) . . . . (PAGE 81)

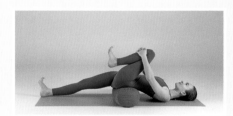

4. Therapeutic Psoas Release
   (5 minutes) . . . . (PAGE 86)

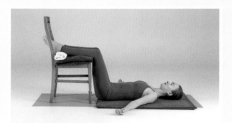

Practice Sequence F: Balancing Scoliosis

Physical Effect: Lengthens and balances spinal asymmetry.

Energetic Effect: Relieves and enlivens.

Practice Time: 60–90 minutes

1. Constructive Rest Position with cross-belt
   (7 minutes) . . . . **(PAGE 49)**

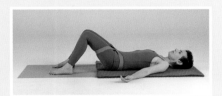

2. Pelvic Reset (5 minutes) . . . . . **(PAGES 133–137)**

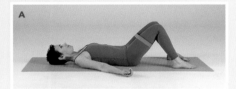

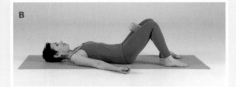

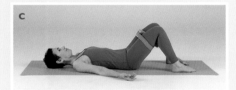

3. Prone Half-Butterfly with MR Ball
   (7 minutes each side) . . . . **(PAGE 64)**

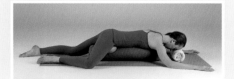

4. Half Bow with Isometric Release
   (*Ardha Dhanurasana*)
   (×5 each side, 5 minutes total) . . . . **(PAGE 78)**

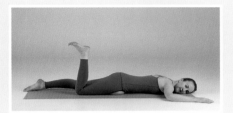

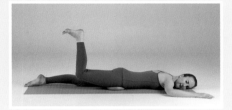

5. Downward Facing Dog
   (*Adho Mukha Svanasana*)
   (×3, 30 seconds–1 minute) . . . . . . **(PAGE 159)**

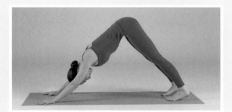

6. Half Dog Pose at Wall
   (*Ardha Adho Mukha Svanasana*)
   (×3, 30 seconds) . . . . **(PAGE 103)**

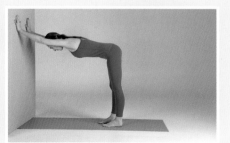

sequence continues on next page ⟶

7. Spinal Release on the Chair, Variation A
(5–7 minutes) . . . . (PAGE 96)

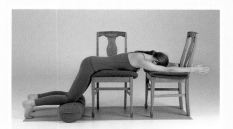

8. Spinal Release on the Chair,
Variation B (3 minutes each side) . . (PAGE 97)

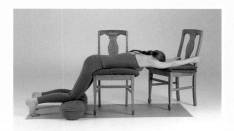

9. Balancing Quadratus Lumborum
(5 minutes each side) . . . . . . (PAGES 98–101)

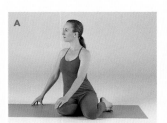

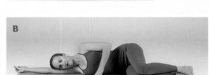

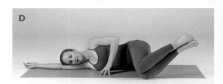

10. Pelvic Reset (5 minutes) . . . (PAGES 133–137)

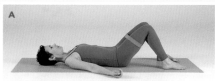

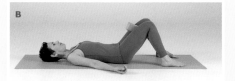

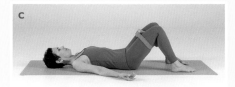

11. Asymmetrical Corpse Pose or Corpse
Pose (*Savasana*)
(5–15 minutes) . . . . (PAGE 101 OR 162)

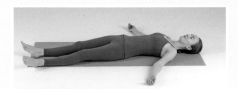

Practice Sequence G: Sacroiliac Discomfort and Sciatica

Physical Effect: Alleviates compression and helps to correct misalignments of the sacroiliac joint. This sequence has been shown to ameliorate symptoms of sciatica.

Energetic Effect: Liberates energy.

Practice Time: 60 minutes

1. Pelvic Reset (5 minutes) . . . . **(PAGES 133–137)**

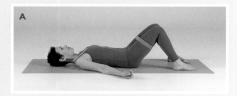

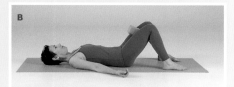

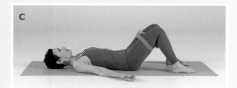

2. Constructive Rest Position with MR Ball (or the variation that provides the greatest sense of release) (7 minutes) . . . . **(PAGE 48)**

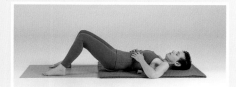

3. Prone Half-Butterfly with MR Ball (7 minutes each side) . . . . **(PAGE 64)**

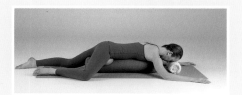

4. Half Bow with Isometric Release (*Ardha Dhanurasana*) (×5 each side, 5 minutes total) . . . . **(PAGE 78)**

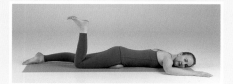

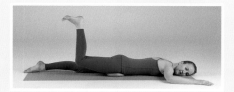

5. Half Reclining Hero's Pose (*Ardha Supta Virasana*) (3 minutes each side) . . . . **(PAGE 155–157)**

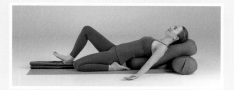

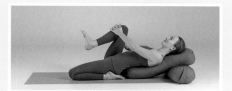

sequence continues on next page ⟶

6. Supine Big Toe Pose
 (*Supta Padangusthasana*)
 (5 minutes each side) . . . . . . **(PAGES 137–141)**

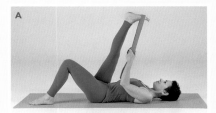

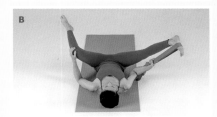

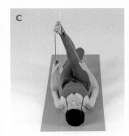
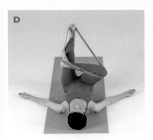

7. Therapeutic Psoas Release
 (5–10 minutes) . . . . **(PAGE 86)**

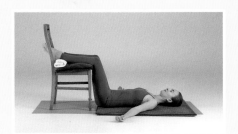

Practice Sequence H:
Weekend Warrior Repair Kit

Physical Effect: Combats muscle stiffness and soreness caused through overexertion.
Energetic Effect: Relieves and relaxes.
Practice Time: 45 minutes

1. Prone Half-Butterfly with MR Ball
   (7 minutes each side) . . . . **(PAGE 64)**

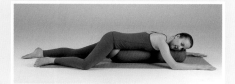

2. Prone Half-Butterfly with Hip Slides
   (5 minutes each side) . . . . **(PAGE 66)**

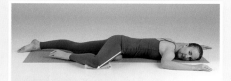

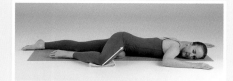

3. Half Bow with Isometric Release
   (*Ardha Dhanurasana*)
   (×5 each side, 5 minutes total) . . . . **(PAGE 78)**

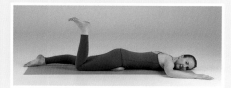

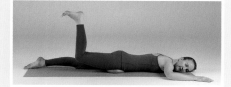

4. Releasing the Psoas on a Bolster or
   Thunderbolt Variation with a Partner
   (1 minute each side) . . . . **(PAGES 81–82)**

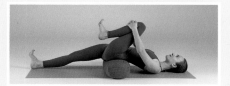

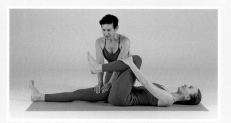

5. Half Reclining Hero's Pose, Variation B
   (*Ardha Supta Virasana*)
   (3 minutes each side) . . . . **(PAGE 157)**

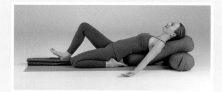

6. Downward Facing Dog
   (*Adho Mukha Svanasana*)
   (×3, 30 seconds–1 minute) . . . . . . **(PAGE 159)**

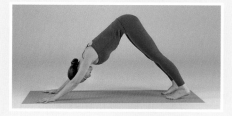

7. Therapeutic Psoas Release
   (5 minutes) . . . . **(PAGE 86)**

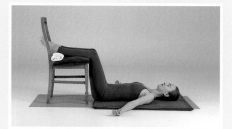

Practice Sequence I:
Relieving Low Back Pain

Physical Effect: Soothes and releases the psoas and spinal muscles.

Energetic Effect: Relieves and relaxes.

Practice Time: 30–35 minutes

1. Constructive Rest Position combined with Abdominal Breathing (hands resting on lower abdomen) (5 minutes) . . . . **(PAGE 48)**

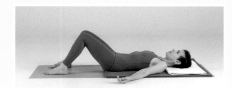

2. Pelvic Reset (5 minutes) . . . . **(PAGES 133–137)**

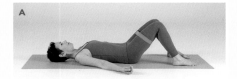

3. Prone Half-Butterfly with MR Ball (5 minutes each side) . . . . **(PAGE 64)**

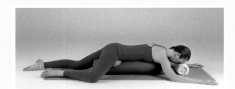

4. Lengthening the Psoas, Variation A (3 minutes each side) . . . . **(PAGE 75)**

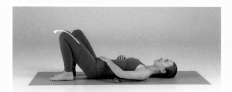

5. Pelvic Reset (5 minutes) . . . . . **(PAGES 133–137)**

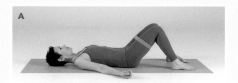
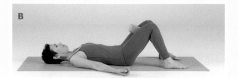
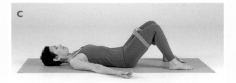

6. Low Bridge Pose, Variation A (*Setu Bandhasana*) (×8) (2 minutes) . . . . **(PAGE 125)**

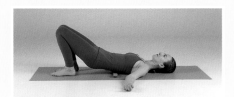

7. The Great Rejuvenator (*Viparita Karani*) (5–10 minutes) . . . . **(PAGES 129–130)**

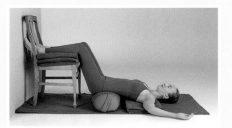

Chapter Notes

CHAPTER ONE

1. Werner Kahle, Helmut Leonhardt, and Werner Platzer, *Color Atlas and Textbook of Human Anatomy, Volume 1: Locomotor System*, Thieme Medical Publishers, Chicago and London, 1978.
2. Janet Travell and David Simon, *Myofascial Pain and Dysfunction: Lower Extremities Volume 2*, 1st edition, Williams & Wilkins, Baltimore, MD, 1993, page 89.
3. Muscle Release Balls (MR Balls) are small, *very soft* plastic balls that can be used in myriad ways to support the body. Ideally, the balls used in our exercises should be no bigger than 23 centimeters (9 inches). MR Balls can be inflated or deflated depending on the specific exercise and the needs of your structure. Whenever they are used under the pelvis, they must be at least 50 percent deflated. Many of the soft balls at toy stores are unsuitable for this therapeutic work. Therefore, we advise specifically sourcing our MR Ball to ensure that you get the best results. www.MyMRBall.com
4. Karlfried Graf Dürckheim, *Hara: The Vital Center of Man*, 4th edition, Inner Traditions, Rochester, VT, 2004.
5. Philip Shepherd, *New Self, New World: Recovering Our Senses in The Twenty-First Century*, North Atlantic Books, Berkeley, CA, 2010.
6. An interview, by Amnon Buchbinder, "Out of Our Heads: Philip Shepherd on the Brain in Our Belly," *The Sun Magazine*, April 2013, http://thesunmagazine.org/issues/448/out_of_our_heads.
7. Michael D. Gershon, M.D., *The Second Brain*, Harper, New York, 1998.

CHAPTER TWO

1. Many traditional anatomy books do not include the two ilium of the pelvis as part of the axial skeleton. Because so many Yoga injuries are caused through hypermobility between the sacrum and ilium, we feel that one of the first steps in correcting this dysfunction is to consider the pelvis as one cohesive unit.
2. S. G. T. Gibbons, B. Pelley, and J. Molgaard, "Biomechanics and Stability Mechanisms of Psoas Major," *Proceedings of the Fourth Interdisciplinary World Congress on Low Back Pain*, November 9–11, Montreal, Canada, 2001.
3. Thomas Myers, *Anatomy Trains*, Churchill Livingstone, New York, 2001.
4. Patrick Hanson, S. Peter Magnusson, Henrik Sorensen, and Erik B. Simonsen, "Anatomical Differences in Psoas Muscles in Young Black and White Men," *Journal of Anatomy* 194, pt. 2 (1999): 303–307. Autopsies of black and white men showed that only 9 percent of black subjects had a psoas minor compared with 87 percent in white subjects. Furthermore, the psoas major in black subjects was almost four times that of the white subjects, with the size of psoas major being calculated from cross-sectional analysis. In general, the size of a muscle is often an indicator of its strength. This study suggests that there may be racial differences in anatomical morphology that could contribute to higher or lower incidences of spinal pathology such as disk herniation. A larger psoas major also might contribute to greater strength in activities such as running.
5. Seen in cross-section, the fibers from the higher levels of the spine form the outer surface of the muscle and those from the lower levels of the spine form the deeper substance of the muscle.
6. Thomas Myers, *Anatomy Trains*, Churchill Livingstone, New York, 2001.
7. Thomas Myers, "The Opinioned Psoas, Part 2," *Massage & Bodywork Magazine*, April/May 2001.
8. M. Yoshio, G. Murakami, T. Sato, S. Sato, and S. Noriyasu, "The Function of Psoas Major Muscle: Passive Kinetics and Morphological Studies Using Donated Cadavers," *Journal of Orthopedic Science* 7, no. 2 (2002): 199–207.
9. Nikolai Bogduk, *Clinical and Radiological Anatomy of*

the Lumbar Spine, 5th edition, Elsevier Churchill Livingstone, London, 2012.

10. Ida P. Rolf, *Rolfing: The Integration of Human Structures*, Harper & Row, New York, 1977.

11. Mabel Todd, *The Thinking Body*, Princeton Book Company, New Jersey, 1980. (This is a new edition of the original publication which first appeared in 1937.)

12. S. G. T. Gibbons, B. Pelley, and J. Molgaard, "Biomechanics and Stability Mechanisms of Psoas Major," *Proceedings of the Fourth Interdisciplinary World Congress on Low Back Pain*, Montreal Canada, November 9–11, 2001.

13. T. Sato and M. Hashimoto, "Morphological Analysis of the Fascial Lamination of the Trunk," *Bulletin of Tokyo Medical and Dental University* 31, no. 1 (1984): 21–32.

14. Robert Schleip, "Adventures in the Jungle of Neuro-Myofascial Net," *Rolf Lines*, May 1996.

15. Robert Schleip, Thomas W. Findley, Leon Chaitow, and Peter A. Huijing, eds., *Fascia: The Tensional Network of the Human Body*, 1st edition, Churchill Livingston, London, 2012.

16. Ana R. C. Donati, et al., "Long-Term Training with a Brain-Machine Interface-Based Gait Protocol Induces Partial Neurological Recovery in Paraplegic Patients," *Scientific Reports* 6 (2016): 30383.

17. Clare Raffety, Certified Anusara Yoga Teacher (2004–2012), Restorative Yoga Teacher (Judith Lasater Certified), Yoga Australia Registered Level 3 Teacher, www.yogafromtheheart.com.au.

18. Andrew P. Thomas, "Yoga and Cardiovascular Function," *Journal of the International Association of Yoga Therapists* 4, no. 1 (1993): 39–42.

19. J. Van Dixhoorn, "Relaxation Therapy in Cardiac Rehabilitation," *Den Haag: Doninklijke Bibliotheek*, 1990.

20. A. Hymes and P. Nuernberger, "Breathing Patterns Found in Heart Attack Patients," *Research Bulletin of the Himalayan International Institute* 2, no. 2 (1980): 10–12.

21. Ida P. Rolf, *Rolfing: The Integration of Human Structures*, Harper & Row, New York, 1977.

22. Mohammad Diab, *Lexicon of Orthopaedic Etymology*, Amsterdam, Harwood Academic Publishers, 1999.

23. R. C. Schafer and Leonard Faye, *Motion Palpation*, 2nd edition, The Motion Palpation Institute & ACA Press, Huntington Beach, CA, 1990, chapter 6.

24. Karlfried Graf Dürckheim, *Hara: The Vital Center of Man*, 4th edition, Inner Traditions, Rochester, VT, 2004, pages 84–85.

CHAPTER THREE

1. David H. Coulter, *Anatomy of Hatha Yoga,* Body and Breath, Inc., Honesdale, Pennsylvania, 2001. Coulter refers more accurately to this type of breathing as Thoraco-Diaphragmatic Breathing. For simplicity, we have abbreviated it to Diaphragmatic Breathing.

2. For more information on Diaphragmatic Breathing, see Donna Farhi, *The Breathing Book*, Henry Holt and Company, New York, 1996.

3. For a more thorough explanation of Ujjayi, see Donna Farhi, *Yoga, Mind, Body & Spirit*, Henry Holt and Company, New York, 2000, pages 33–34.

4. MR Balls are small, *very soft* plastic balls that can be used in myriad ways to support the body. Ideally, the balls used in our exercises should be no bigger than 23 centimeters (9 inches). MR Balls can be inflated or deflated depending on the specific exercise and the needs of your structure. Whenever they are used under the pelvis, they must be at least 50 percent deflated. Many of the soft balls at toy stores are unsuitable for this therapeutic work. Therefore, we advise specifically sourcing our MR Ball to ensure that you get the best results. www.MyMRBall.com

CHAPTER FOUR

1. MR Balls are small, *very soft* plastic balls that can be used in myriad ways to support the body. Ideally, the balls used in our exercises should be no bigger than 23 centimeters (9 inches). MR Balls can be inflated or deflated depending on the specific exercise and the needs of your structure. Whenever they are used under the pelvis, they must be at least 50 percent deflated. Many of the soft balls at toy stores are unsuitable for this therapeutic work. Therefore, we advise specifically sourcing our MR Ball to ensure that you get the best results. www.MyMRBall.com

2. Turning the forearms out helps transfer weight first to the shoulder girdle and then to the spine, reducing the leveraging into the lower lumbar spine. This position also activates the posterior inferior serratus, which stabilizes the vulnerable transition zone between the base of the rib cage and the lumbar spine. The posterior inferior serratus attaches to the spinous processes of T11–L3 via the thoracolumbar fascia (Illustration 25C, page 109). We consider it an accessory muscle to the secondary core muscles.

CHAPTER FIVE

1. Several recent studies have shown a correlation between long hours of sedentary sitting and increased likelihood of death as well as higher levels of health problems, such as type 2 diabetes, strokes, high blood pressure, cardiovascular disease, cancer, and depression. Julie Corliss, "Too Much Sitting Linked to Heart Disease, Diabetes, Premature Death," Harvard Health Blog, January 22, 2015, http://www.health.harvard.edu/blog/much-sitting-linked-heart-disease-diabetes-premature-death-201501227618.

2. MR Balls are small, *very soft* plastic balls that can be used in myriad ways to support the body. Ideally, the balls used in our exercises should be no bigger than 23 centimeters (9 inches). MR Balls can be inflated or deflated depending on the specific exercise and the needs of your structure. Whenever they are used under the pelvis, they must be at least 50 percent deflated. Many of the soft balls at toy stores are unsuitable for this therapeutic work. Therefore, we advise specifically sourcing our MR Ball to ensure that you get the best results. www.MyMRBall.com

3. Isometric exercise is a form of exercise involving the static contraction of a muscle without any visible movement in the angle of the joint. This is reflected in the name; the term "isometric" combines the Greek the prefixes "iso" (same) with "metric" (distance), meaning that in these exercises, the length of the muscle and the angle of the joint do not change. It often is used in strength training regimens.

4. The relationship between the kidneys in the back of the body and the transverse line that runs from the kidneys via the ureters to the bladder is an organic corollary to the psoas muscles, often referred to as the "organic psoas." By visualizing a dynamic tension of the ureters, one can stabilize the spine, especially at the vulnerable bridging point between the base of the rib cage (T12) and the top of the lumbar spine (L1).

5. Experienced teachers can use the arch of the sole of the foot instead of the hands. Face toward your client's feet so that the pressure of your foot assists in giving slight traction to the hip. This adjustment can feel smoother and deeper than using the hands. Begin with light pressure and ask for your client's permission to use deeper pressure.

CHAPTER SIX

1. Structural scoliosis results from a genetic predisposition for uneven bone growth of the vertebral bodies. Functional scoliosis is caused by soft tissue changes, but it can progress to structural scoliosis over time as bone responds to sustained muscular stress.

2. Thomas Hanna, *Somatics*, 1st edition, Addison-Wesley Publishing Company, New York, 1988.

3. Because of the complexity of the rotation of spinal vertebrae, it sometimes may feel even better to move the legs off-center to the right (for right-sided discomfort), but this is the exception to the rule.

CHAPTER SEVEN

1. C. Richardson, G. Jull, P. Hodges, and J. Hides, *Therapeutic Exercise for Spinal Segmental Stabilization in Low Pack Pain: Scientific Basis and Clinical Approach*, Churchill Livingstone, Edinburgh, London, 1999.

2. Sandy Saiko, BOHE, DC, MSc, and Kent Stuber, BSc, DC, MSc, "Psoas Major: A Case Report and Review of Its Anatomy, Biomechanics, and Clinical Implications," *Journal of the Canadian Chiropractic Association* 53, no. 4 (2009): 311–318.

3. S. R. Ward, C. W. Kim, C. M. Eng, et al. "Architectural Analysis and Intraoperative Measurements Demonstrate the Unique Design of the Multifidus Muscle for Lumbar Spine Stability, *Journal of Bone and Joint Surgery* 91 (2009): 176–185.

4. L. A. Danneels, P. L. Coorevits, A. M. Cools, et al., "Differences in Electromyographic Activity in the Multifidus Muscle and Iliocostalis Lumborum between Healthy Subjects and Patients with Subacute and Chronic Low Back Pain," *European Spine Journal* 11, no. 1 (2002): 13–19.

5. "Multifidus Muscle Design Contributes to Spine Stability," News-Medical.net, January 7, 2009, http://www.news-medical.net/news/2009/01/07/44811.aspx.

6. Eric Franklin, *Pelvic Power: Mind/Body Exercises for Strength, Flexibility, Posture and Balance*, Elysian Editions, Princeton Book Company, New Jersey, 2002.

7. Leslie Howard Yoga, lesliehowardyoga.com.

8. MR Balls are small, *very soft* plastic balls that can be used in myriad ways to support the body. Ideally, the balls used in our exercises should be no bigger than 23 centimeters (9 inches). MR Balls can be inflated or deflated depending on the specific exercise and the needs of your structure. Whenever they are used under the pelvis, they must be at least 50 percent deflated. Many of the soft balls at toy stores are unsuitable for this therapeutic work. Therefore, we advise specifically sourcing our MR Ball to ensure that you get the best results. www.MyMRBall.com

9. The concept of the Figure-8 Loop was first introduced to me through the work of Narelle Carter-Quinlan. Further research traced the idea back to

the work of Peggy Hackney (*Making Connections*, Routledge, New York, 1998) and Joan Skinner, but I suspect this imagery also might be present in the work of Qi Gong and Tai Chi practitioners. All ideokinetic images, however, are simply that, "ideas" about movement, and they should be used as a starting point for your own exploration in any way that is relevant to the integration of your own structure. Feel free to change the image and its pathway in any way that works best for you.

10. Your inner ear registers the position of the head relative to the center of the earth. We believe that the *hara* also registers its position relative to the core of the earth and postulate that the inner ear and the abdominal brain communicate with each other to facilitate proprioception of the body.

11. Mary Wanless, *Riding with Your Mind Essentials*, Trafalgar Square Books, North Pomfret, VT, 2002.

12. Sarah Keys, *The Back Sufferers' Bible*, 2nd edition, Allen and Unwin, St. Leonards, NSW, 2012

CHAPTER EIGHT

This chapter does not include notes.

CHAPTER NINE

1. Donna Farhi, *Yoga, Mind, Body & Spirit: A Return to Wholeness*, Henry Holt & Company, New York, 2000 This is a comprehensive guide to Yoga practice that includes "Essential Skills" sections for standing postures, forward bends, back bends, twists, arm balances, inversions, and restorative Yoga.

2. Muscle Release Balls (MR Balls) are small, *very soft* plastic balls that can be used in myriad ways to support the body. Ideally, the balls used in our exercises should be no bigger than 23 centimeters (9 inches). MR Balls can be inflated or deflated depending on the specific exercise and the needs of your structure. Whenever they are used under the pelvis, they must be at least 50 percent deflated. Many of the soft balls at toy stores are unsuitable for this therapeutic work. Therefore, we advise specifically sourcing our MR Ball to ensure that you get the best results. www.MyMRBall.com